KIDNEY DISEASE DIET

FOR SENIORS

ON STAGE 3

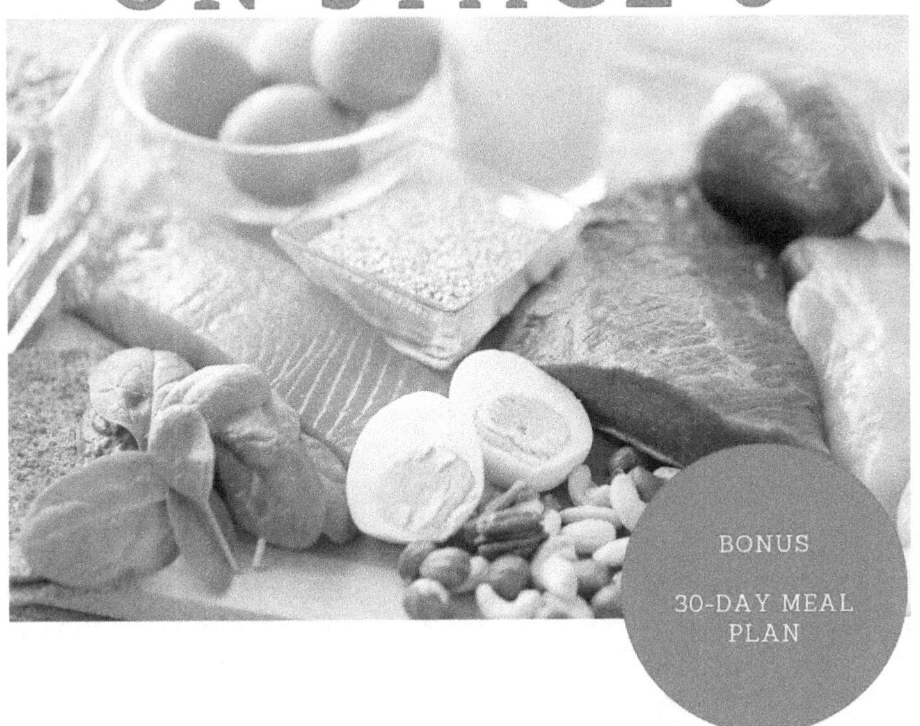

A Senior's Guide to Culinary Health with 180 Easy-to-Prepare and Delicious Recipes Featuring Low Sodium, Low Potassium, Low Phosphorus, and High Flavor

JENNIFER J RODRIGUEZ

KIDNEY DISEASE DIET FOR SENIORS ON STAGE 3

A Senior's Guide to Culinary Health with 180 Easy-to-Prepare and Delicious Recipes Featuring Low Sodium, Low Potassium, Low Phosphorus, and High Flavor

Jennifer J Rodriguez

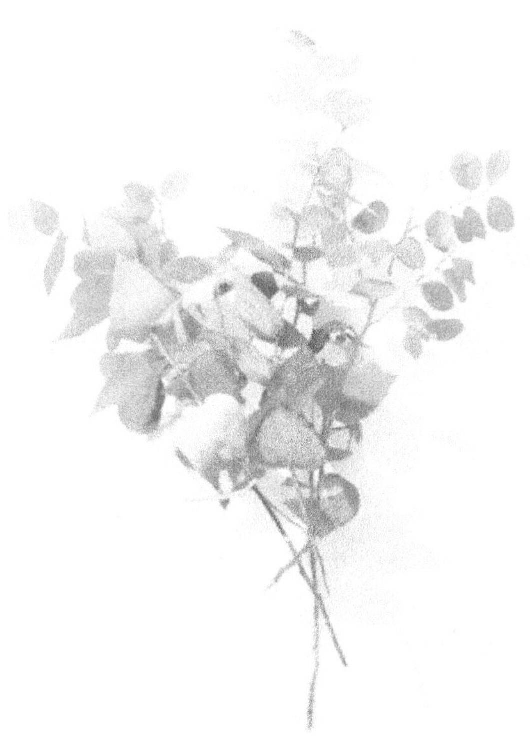

INTRODUCTION

As a registered dietitian nutritionist, I'm deeply committed to helping individuals understand and manage stage 3 kidney disease through proper nutrition.

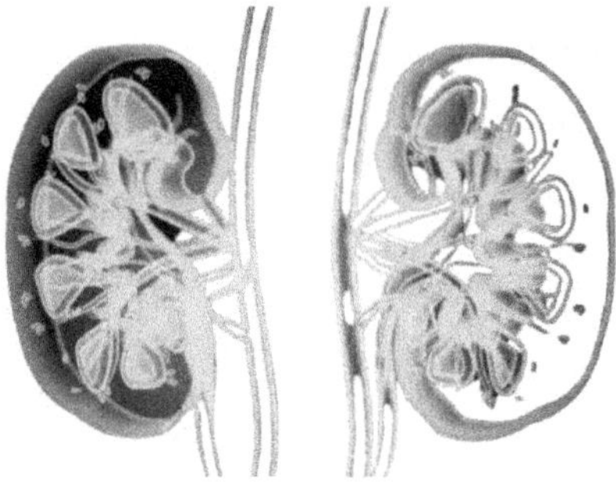

Kidneys play a vital role in filtering waste products and excess fluids from the blood, regulating electrolyte levels, and maintaining overall fluid balance in the body. However, when kidney function becomes impaired, as in stage 3 kidney disease, it's crucial to make dietary adjustments to support kidney function and prevent further deterioration.

Understanding Stage 3 Kidney Disease:

Stage 3 kidney disease signifies a moderate decrease in kidney function, with a glomerular filtration rate (GFR) ranging from 30 to 59 milliliters per minute per 1.73 meters squared.

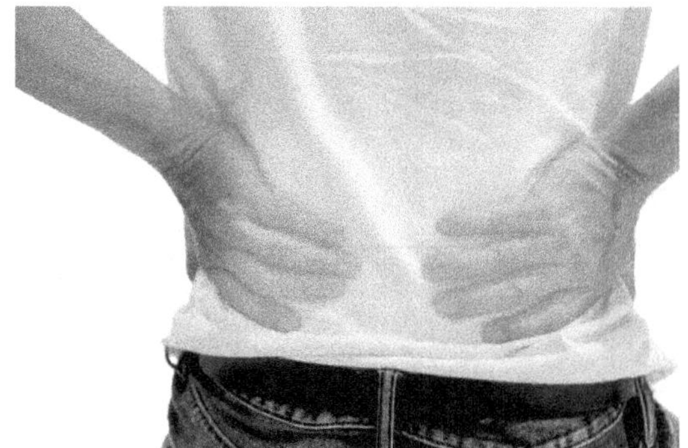

At this stage, individuals may start to experience symptoms such as fatigue, fluid retention, changes in urine output, and electrolyte imbalances. It's essential to recognize the significance of early intervention through lifestyle modifications, including dietary changes, to slow the progression of kidney disease and minimize complications.

Importance of Diet in Managing Kidney Health

Diet plays a pivotal role in managing stage 3 kidney disease by helping to alleviate symptoms, maintain optimal nutritional status, and delay the need for dialysis or transplantation.

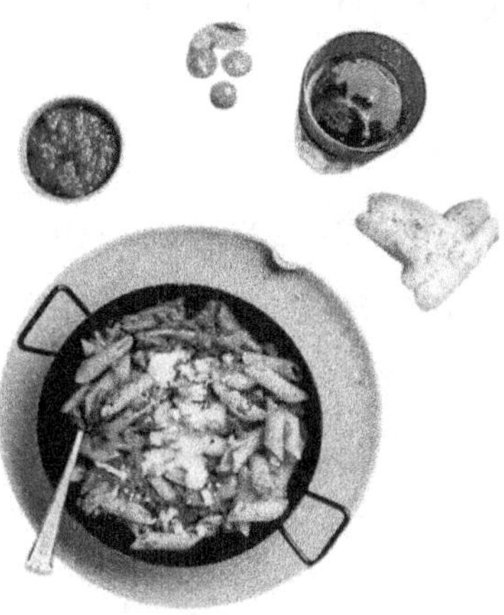

A kidney-friendly diet focuses on reducing the workload on the kidneys, limiting the intake of certain nutrients that can burden the kidneys, such as sodium, potassium, phosphorus, and protein, while ensuring an adequate intake of essential nutrients. By following a well-balanced and individualized meal plan, individuals with stage 3 kidney disease can better manage their condition and improve their overall quality of life.

Tips for Adhering to Dietary Restrictions

Adhering to dietary restrictions can be challenging, but with proper guidance and support, it's entirely achievable. Here are some practical tips to help individuals with stage 3 kidney disease adhere to their dietary restrictions:

1. Work with a Registered Dietitian: A registered dietitian specialized in kidney health can provide personalized nutrition counseling and develop a customized meal plan tailored to individual needs, preferences, and medical conditions.

2. Read Food Labels: Familiarize yourself with reading food labels to identify high sodium, potassium, phosphorus, and protein content in packaged foods. Choose low-sodium and phosphorus-free alternatives whenever possible.

3. Monitor Portion Sizes: Controlling portion sizes is crucial, especially for foods high in potassium and phosphorus. Use measuring cups, spoons, or a food scale to accurately portion out foods and prevent overconsumption.

4. Incorporate Variety: Embrace variety in your diet by including a wide range of fruits, vegetables, whole grains, lean proteins, and healthy fats. Experiment with different cooking methods and flavor-enhancing herbs and spices to keep meals interesting and enjoyable.

5. Stay Hydrated: Adequate hydration is essential for kidney health. Aim to drink plenty of fluids throughout the day, primarily water. Limit the intake of high-calorie and sugary beverages, as well as those containing phosphorus additives.

6. Plan Ahead: Plan your meals and snacks in advance to ensure you have kidney-friendly options readily available. Batch cooking and meal prepping can save time and make sticking to your dietary plan more convenient.

7. Seek Support: Joining a support group or connecting with others who are also managing kidney disease can provide valuable encouragement, tips, and resources for navigating dietary restrictions and maintaining motivation.

CHAPTER 1

SENIOR-FRIENDLY KITCHEN ESSENTIALS

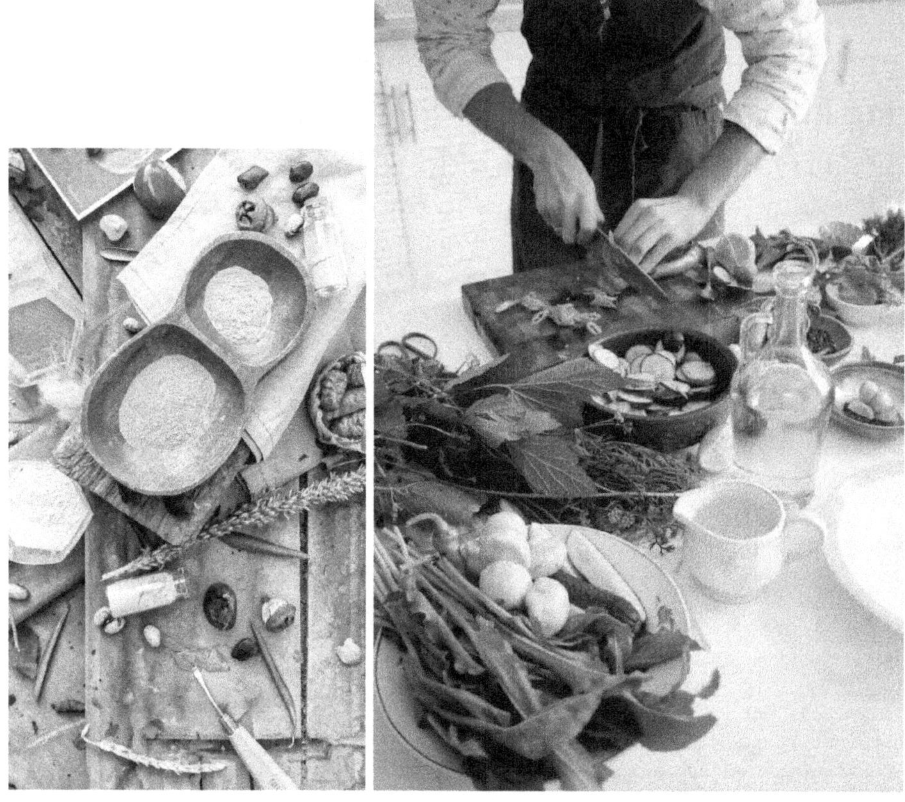

I understand the vital role that a well-equipped kitchen plays in supporting the dietary needs of older adults, especially those managing conditions like stage 3 kidney disease. Senior-friendly kitchen essentials encompass not only the tools and equipment necessary for preparing nutritious meals but also the strategic stocking of pantry items and smart shopping practices tailored to the unique needs of older individuals. In this section, I'll delve into each aspect, offering valuable insights and practical tips to empower seniors to create delicious, kidney-friendly meals at home while optimizing their health and well-being.

Must-Have Tools and Equipment

1. Quality Knives: Invest in a set of sharp, comfortable knives to make meal preparation safer and more efficient. Opt for knives with ergonomic handles to reduce strain on aging hands.

2. Non-Slip Cutting Boards: Choose cutting boards with non-slip surfaces to prevent accidents in the kitchen. Consider boards with bright colors to enhance visibility for seniors with visual impairments.

3. Easy-Grip Utensils: Look for utensils with larger, ergonomic handles that are easier for seniors to grasp and manipulate. Silicone-coated utensils provide a non-slip grip and are gentle on arthritic hands.

4. Adaptive Kitchen Gadgets: Explore adaptive kitchen gadgets designed specifically for seniors or individuals with mobility issues, such as jar openers, easy-twist can openers, and one-handed cutting tools.

5. Adjustable Height Kitchen Tools: Consider adjustable-height countertops, cabinets, and shelving to accommodate seniors with mobility challenges or wheelchair users, ensuring accessibility and safety in the kitchen.

6. Electric Appliances: Simplify meal preparation with electric appliances like slow cookers, pressure cookers, and electric kettles, which offer convenience and ease of use for seniors.

7. Microwave with Easy Controls: Choose a microwave with large, user-friendly buttons and intuitive controls for seniors with cognitive impairments or limited dexterity.

8. Safety Features: Install safety features such as grab bars, anti-scald devices, and smoke detectors with strobe lights and alarms to enhance kitchen safety for seniors.

Stocking Your Pantry for Success

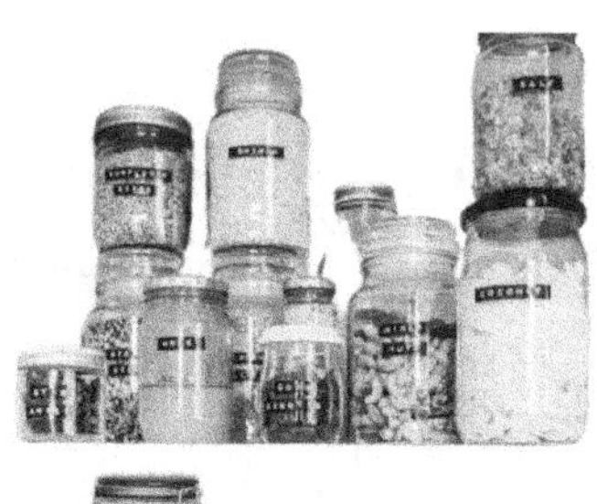

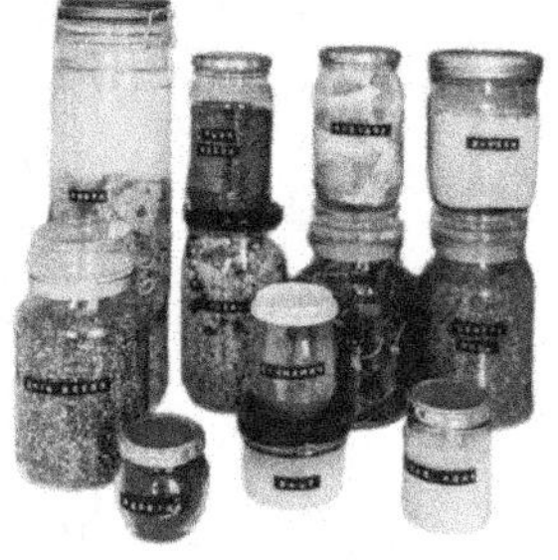

1. Low-Sodium Broths and Stocks: Opt for low-sodium broths and stocks as the foundation for soups, stews, and sauces, reducing sodium intake without compromising flavor.

2. Canned Beans and Legumes: Keep a variety of canned beans and legumes on hand for quick and convenient sources of plant-based protein, fiber, and essential nutrients.

3. Whole Grains: Stock up on whole grains such as brown rice, quinoa, oats, and whole wheat pasta to provide sustained energy and promote heart health.

4. Herbs and Spices: Enhance flavor without adding extra salt by incorporating a diverse array of herbs and spices into your pantry, including basil, oregano, turmeric, and cinnamon.

5. Low-Potassium Fruits and Vegetables: Choose low-potassium options like apples, berries, cabbage, cauliflower, and green beans to support kidney health while adding color and variety to your meals.

6. Healthy Cooking Oils: Opt for heart-healthy oils such as olive oil, avocado oil, and canola oil for cooking and salad dressings, providing essential fatty acids without excess saturated or trans fats.

7. Low-Phosphorus Dairy Alternatives: Select low-phosphorus dairy alternatives such as almond milk, coconut milk, and rice milk to minimize phosphorus intake while still enjoying dairy-free beverages.

8. Sugar-Free Sweeteners: Use sugar-free sweeteners like stevia, monk fruit, or erythritol to sweeten beverages, desserts, and baked goods without impacting blood sugar levels.

Smart Shopping Strategies for Seniors

1. Plan Meals in Advance: Create a weekly meal plan and shopping list to streamline grocery shopping and ensure you have all the necessary ingredients on hand.

2. Shop the Perimeter: Focus on purchasing fresh produce, lean proteins, and dairy products from the perimeter of the grocery store, where the majority of whole, nutrient-dense foods are located.

3. Read Labels Carefully: Pay close attention to food labels, particularly the sodium, potassium, and phosphorus content, to make informed choices that align with your dietary restrictions and kidney health goals.

4. Choose Frozen and Canned Options Wisely: Opt for frozen or canned fruits and vegetables without added salt or sugar to minimize food waste and maximize convenience without sacrificing nutritional quality.

5. Buy in Bulk and Freeze Portions: Take advantage of bulk purchasing for non-perishable items like grains, beans, and spices, and portion them into freezer-safe containers for long-term storage and convenience.

6. Utilize Online Shopping Services: Explore online grocery delivery or pickup services for added convenience, especially for seniors with limited mobility or transportation options.

7. Take Advantage of Senior Discounts: Look for stores that offer senior discounts or special savings days to stretch your grocery budget further and make healthy eating more affordable.

Chapter 2

Nourishing Breakfast Recipes

Welcome to the Nourishing Breakfast Recipes section of our kidney disease diet cookbook tailored for seniors in stage 3. I am thrilled to share with you a variety of delicious and nutrient-rich breakfast options designed to support your overall well-being.

Breakfast is often referred to as the most important meal of the day, and for good reason. It provides the body with essential nutrients and energy to kick-start metabolism and fuel daily activities. For seniors managing stage 3 kidney disease, it's crucial to choose breakfast options that are not only delicious but also kidney-friendly, supporting optimal health and managing kidney function.

Energizing Morning Meals

1. Protein-Packed Breakfast Burrito Bowl

Ingredients:

- 1 cup cooked quinoa

- 1/2 cup black beans, drained and rinsed

- 1/4 cup diced tomatoes

- 1/4 cup diced bell peppers

- 1/4 cup diced avocado

- 2 eggs, scrambled

- Salt and pepper, to taste

- Optional toppings: salsa, Greek yogurt, chopped cilantro

Instructions:

1. In a skillet over medium heat, warm the cooked quinoa and black beans until heated through.

2. Divide the quinoa and black bean mixture into two bowls.

3. Top each bowl with scrambled eggs, diced tomatoes, bell peppers, and avocado.

4. Season with salt and pepper to taste.

5. Serve with optional toppings such as salsa, Greek yogurt, and chopped cilantro.

Cooking Time: 15 minutes

Nutritional Information (per serving):

- Calories: 350

- Protein: 18g

- Carbohydrates: 35g

- Fat: 16g

- Fiber: 8g

2. Greek Yogurt Parfait with Fresh Berries and Almonds

Ingredients:

- 1 cup plain Greek yogurt

- 1/2 cup mixed fresh berries (such as strawberries, blueberries, raspberries)

- 2 tablespoons sliced almonds

- 1 tablespoon honey (optional)

Instructions:

1. In a glass or bowl, layer Greek yogurt, mixed berries, and sliced almonds.

2. Drizzle with honey if desired.

3. Serve immediately.

Preparation Time: 5 minutes

Nutritional Information (per serving):

- Calories: 250

- Protein: 20g

- Carbohydrates: 20g

- Fat: 10g

- Fiber: 5g

3. Spinach and Feta Omelette Roll-Ups

Ingredients:

- 2 large eggs

- 1 tablespoon milk

- 1/4 cup fresh spinach leaves

- 2 tablespoons crumbled feta cheese

- Salt and pepper, to taste

- Cooking spray

Instructions:

1. In a small bowl, whisk together eggs and milk. Season with salt and pepper.

2. Heat a non-stick skillet over medium heat and lightly coat with cooking spray.

3. Pour the egg mixture into the skillet and swirl to coat the bottom evenly.

4. Cook until the edges start to set, about 1-2 minutes.

5. Sprinkle spinach and feta cheese evenly over the omelette.

6. Using a spatula, gently roll the omelette into a tight cylinder.

7. Remove from heat and let it sit for a minute before slicing into pieces.

8. Serve immediately.

Cooking Time: 5 minutes

Nutritional Information (per serving):

- Calories: 200

- Protein: 15g

- Carbohydrates: 2g

- Fat: 14g

- Fiber: 1g

4. Quinoa Breakfast Bowl with Roasted Vegetables

Ingredients:

- 1/2 cup cooked quinoa

- 1 cup mixed roasted vegetables (such as bell peppers, zucchini, and cherry tomatoes)

- 1 tablespoon olive oil

- Salt and pepper, to taste

- 2 eggs, poached or fried

- Optional toppings: chopped fresh herbs, avocado slices

Instructions:

1. Preheat the oven to 400°F (200°C).

2. Toss the mixed vegetables with olive oil, salt, and pepper on a baking sheet.

3. Roast in the preheated oven for 15-20 minutes, or until tender and slightly caramelized.

4. In a bowl, layer cooked quinoa and roasted vegetables.

5. Top with poached or fried eggs.

6. Garnish with optional toppings such as chopped fresh herbs and avocado slices.

7. Serve immediately.

Cooking Time: 30 minutes

Nutritional Information (per serving):

- Calories: 400

- Protein: 18g

- Carbohydrates: 30g

- Fat: 24g

- Fiber: 7g

5. Smoked Salmon and Avocado Toast

Ingredients:

- 2 slices whole grain bread, toasted

- 1/2 avocado, mashed

- 2 ounces smoked salmon

- 1 tablespoon capers

- Lemon wedges, for serving

- Fresh dill or parsley, for garnish (optional)

Instructions:

1. Spread mashed avocado evenly onto toasted whole grain bread slices.

2. Top each slice with smoked salmon.

3. Sprinkle capers over the salmon.

4. Serve with lemon wedges on the side.

5. Garnish with fresh dill or parsley if desired.

6. Serve immediately.

Preparation Time: 10 minutes

Nutritional Information (per serving):

- Calories: 300

- Protein: 20g

- Carbohydrates: 20g

- Fat: 15g

- Fiber: 8g

6. Banana Nut Overnight Oats

Ingredients:

- 1/2 cup rolled oats

- 1/2 cup unsweetened almond milk (or milk of choice)

- 1/2 ripe banana, mashed

- 1 tablespoon chopped walnuts

- 1 tablespoon honey or maple syrup

- 1/2 teaspoon ground cinnamon

- Pinch of salt

Instructions:

1. In a jar or bowl, combine rolled oats, almond milk, mashed banana, chopped walnuts, honey or maple syrup, cinnamon, and salt.

2. Stir well to combine.

3. Cover and refrigerate overnight, or for at least 4 hours.

4. In the morning, give the oats a stir and add more almond milk if desired for consistency.

5. Serve cold, or warm in the microwave if preferred.

6. Optional: Top with additional sliced banana and a sprinkle of cinnamon before serving.

Preparation Time: 5 minutes (+ overnight chilling)

Nutritional Information (per serving):

- Calories: 300

- Protein: 7g

- Carbohydrates: 50g

- Fat: 9g

- Fiber: 7g

7. Vegetable Frittata Muffins

Ingredients:

- 6 large eggs

- 1/4 cup milk (or milk alternative)

- 1 cup chopped mixed vegetables (such as bell peppers, spinach, onions)

- 1/4 cup shredded cheese (such as cheddar or mozzarella)

- Salt and pepper, to taste

- Cooking spray

Instructions:

1. Preheat the oven to 350°F (175°C) and lightly grease a muffin tin with cooking spray.

2. In a mixing bowl, whisk together eggs, milk, salt, and pepper.

3. Stir in chopped vegetables and shredded cheese.

4. Pour the egg mixture evenly into the prepared muffin tin.

5. Bake for 20-25 minutes, or until the frittata muffins are set and lightly golden on top.

6. Allow to cool slightly before removing from the muffin tin.

7. Serve warm or at room temperature.

Cooking Time: 25 minutes

Nutritional Information (per serving, based on 2 muffins):

- Calories: 200

- Protein: 14g

- Carbohydrates: 5g

- Fat: 14g

- Fiber: 1g

8. Sweet Potato and Black Bean Hash

Ingredients:

- 2 medium sweet potatoes, peeled and diced

- 1 can (15 ounces) black beans, drained and rinsed

- 1 red bell pepper, diced

- 1 small onion, diced

- 2 cloves garlic, minced

- 1 teaspoon ground cumin

- 1/2 teaspoon paprika

- Salt and pepper, to taste

- 2 tablespoons olive oil

- Fresh cilantro, for garnish (optional)

Instructions:

1. Heat olive oil in a large skillet over medium heat.

2. Add diced sweet potatoes and cook until slightly softened, about 5 minutes.

3. Add diced onion, bell pepper, and minced garlic to the skillet. Cook until vegetables are tender, about 5-7 minutes.

4. Stir in black beans, ground cumin, paprika, salt, and pepper. Cook for another 2-3 minutes to heat through.

5. Remove from heat and garnish with fresh cilantro if desired.

6. Serve hot as a hearty breakfast hash.

Cooking Time: 20 minutes

Nutritional Information (per serving):

- Calories: 250

- Protein: 8g

- Carbohydrates: 40g

- Fat: 6g

- Fiber: 9g

9. Chia Seed Pudding with Mango and Coconut

Ingredients:

- 1/4 cup chia seeds

- 1 cup unsweetened coconut milk (or milk of choice)

- 1 tablespoon honey or maple syrup

- 1/2 teaspoon vanilla extract

- 1 ripe mango, diced

- 2 tablespoons shredded coconut

Instructions:

1. In a bowl, whisk together chia seeds, coconut milk, honey or maple syrup, and vanilla extract.

2. Cover and refrigerate for at least 2 hours, or overnight, until the mixture thickens and forms a pudding-like consistency.

3. Once the chia pudding is set, stir well and divide into serving cups or bowls.

4. Top with diced mango and shredded coconut.

5. Serve chilled.

Preparation Time: 5 minutes (+ chilling time)

Nutritional Information (per serving):

- Calories: 250

- Protein: 4g

- Carbohydrates: 30g

- Fat: 13g

- Fiber: 10g

10. Turkey Sausage and Egg Breakfast Sandwich

Ingredients:

- 2 whole grain English muffins, split and toasted

- 4 turkey sausage patties, cooked

- 2 large eggs, fried or scrambled

- 2 slices reduced-fat cheddar cheese

- Salt and pepper, to taste

- Optional toppings: avocado slices, tomato slices, spinach leaves

Instructions:

1. Cook turkey sausage patties according to package instructions.

2. Cook eggs to your preference (fried or scrambled), seasoning with salt and pepper.

3. Assemble the breakfast sandwiches by placing a turkey sausage patty, cooked egg, and slice of cheddar cheese on each toasted English muffin half.

4. Add optional toppings such as avocado slices, tomato slices, and spinach leaves if desired.

5. Serve immediately.

Cooking Time: 10 minutes

Nutritional Information (per serving):

- Calories: 350

- Protein: 25g

- Carbohydrates: 25g

- Fat: 15g

- Fiber: 4g

Delicious Smoothies and Juices

1. Berry Blast Smoothie with Spinach and Flaxseed:

Ingredients:
- 1 cup frozen mixed berries
- 1 cup fresh spinach leaves
- 1 tablespoon ground flaxseed
- 1/2 cup plain Greek yogurt
- 1/2 cup almond milk
- 1 tablespoon honey (optional)
- Ice cubes (optional)

Instructions:
1. In a blender, combine the frozen mixed berries, fresh spinach leaves, ground flaxseed, Greek yogurt, almond milk, and honey (if using).
2. Blend on high until smooth and creamy, adding ice cubes if desired for a colder consistency.
3. Pour into glasses and serve immediately.

Time Frame: Preparation time: 5 minutes

Nutritional Information (per serving):

- Calories: 180 kcal
- Protein: 12g
- Carbohydrates: 25g
- Fat: 5g
- Fiber: 7g

2. Tropical Paradise Smoothie with Pineapple and Coconut Water:

Ingredients:
- 1 cup frozen pineapple chunks
- 1/2 ripe banana
- 1/2 cup coconut water
- 1/2 cup unsweetened coconut milk
- 1 tablespoon shredded coconut (optional)
- Ice cubes (optional)

Instructions:
1. In a blender, combine the frozen pineapple chunks, ripe banana, coconut water, and coconut milk.
2. Add shredded coconut if desired for extra flavor.
3. Blend until smooth and creamy, adding ice cubes if desired for a colder consistency.
4. Pour into glasses and serve immediately.

Time Frame: Preparation time: 5 minutes

Nutritional Information (per serving):
- Calories: 180 kcal
- Protein: 2g
- Carbohydrates: 35g
- Fat: 6g
- Fiber: 5g

3. Green Goddess Smoothie with Kale and Avocado:

Ingredients:
- 1 cup kale leaves, stemmed and chopped
- 1/2 ripe avocado
- 1/2 cup frozen mango chunks
- 1/2 cup green grapes
- 1/2 cup coconut water
- Juice of 1/2 lime
- Ice cubes (optional)

Instructions:
1. In a blender, combine the kale leaves, ripe avocado, frozen mango chunks, green grapes, coconut water, and lime juice.
2. Blend until smooth and creamy, adding ice cubes if desired for a colder consistency.
3. Pour into glasses and serve immediately.

Time Frame: Preparation time: 5 minutes

Nutritional Information (per serving):
- Calories: 200 kcal
- Protein: 3g
- Carbohydrates: 30g
- Fat: 9g
- Fiber: 7g

4. Creamy Mango Lassi Smoothie:

Ingredients:
- 1 cup ripe mango chunks

- 1/2 cup plain Greek yogurt
- 1/2 cup almond milk
- 1 tablespoon honey (optional)
- 1/4 teaspoon ground cardamom
- Ice cubes (optional)

Instructions:

1. In a blender, combine the ripe mango chunks, Greek yogurt, almond milk, honey (if using), and ground cardamom.
2. Blend until smooth and creamy, adding ice cubes if desired for a colder consistency.
3. Pour into glasses and serve immediately.

Time Frame: Preparation time: 5 minutes

Nutritional Information (per serving):
- Calories: 180 kcal
- Protein: 8g
- Carbohydrates: 30g
- Fat: 4g
- Fiber: 3g

5. Citrus Sunrise Juice with Oranges and Carrots:

Ingredients:
- 2 large oranges, peeled and segmented
- 2 large carrots, peeled and chopped
- 1/2 inch piece of ginger, peeled
- 1/2 cup water
- Ice cubes (optional)

Instructions:

1. In a juicer, process the oranges, carrots, and ginger.
2. Add water to dilute the juice to your desired consistency.
3. Serve immediately over ice cubes if desired.

Time Frame: Preparation time: 5 minutes

Nutritional Information (per serving):
- Calories: 120 kcal
- Protein: 2g
- Carbohydrates: 28g
- Fat: 1g
- Fiber: 7g

6. Beet and Berry Booster Smoothie:

Ingredients:
- 1 small beet, peeled and chopped
- 1/2 cup frozen mixed berries
- 1/2 cup plain Greek yogurt
- 1/2 cup almond milk
- 1 tablespoon honey (optional)
- Ice cubes (optional)

Instructions:
1. In a blender, combine the chopped beet, frozen mixed berries, Greek yogurt, almond milk, and honey (if using).
2. Blend until smooth and creamy, adding ice cubes if desired for a colder consistency.
3. Pour into glasses and serve immediately.

Time Frame: Preparation time: 5 minutes

Nutritional Information (per serving):
- Calories: 180 kcal
- Protein: 10g
- Carbohydrates: 25g
- Fat: 4g
- Fiber: 7g

7. Pineapple Cucumber Refresher Juice:

Ingredients:
- 1 cup chopped pineapple
- 1/2 cucumber, peeled and chopped
- 1/2 cup water
- Juice of 1 lime
- Ice cubes (optional)
- Mint leaves for garnish (optional)

Instructions:
1. In a juicer, process the chopped pineapple and cucumber.
2. Add water and lime juice to dilute the juice to your desired consistency.
3. Serve immediately over ice cubes and garnish with mint leaves if desired.

Time Frame: Preparation time: 5 minutes

Nutritional Information (per serving):
- Calories: 90 kcal
- Protein: 1g
- Carbohydrates: 25g
- Fat: 0g
- Fiber: 3g

8. Chocolate Banana Protein Smoothie:

Ingredients:
- 1 ripe banana
- 1 tablespoon unsweetened cocoa powder
- 1 scoop chocolate protein powder
- 1 cup almond milk
- 1 tablespoon almond butter
- Ice cubes (optional)

Instructions:
1. In a blender, combine the ripe banana, cocoa powder, chocolate protein powder, almond milk, and almond butter.
2. Blend until smooth and creamy, adding ice cubes if desired for a colder consistency.
3. Pour into glasses and serve immediately.

Time Frame: Preparation time: 5 minutes

Nutritional Information (per serving):
- Calories: 250 kcal
- Protein: 20g
- Carbohydrates: 30g
- Fat: 8g
- Fiber: 6g

9. Peachy Keen Smoothie with Greek Yogurt:

Ingredients:
- 1 cup frozen peach slices
- 1/2 cup plain Greek yogurt
- 1/2 cup almond milk
- 1 tablespoon honey (optional)

- 1/4 teaspoon vanilla extract
- Ice cubes (optional)

Instructions:

1. In a blender, combine the frozen peach slices, Greek yogurt, almond milk, honey (if using), and vanilla extract.
2. Blend until smooth and creamy, adding ice cubes if desired for a colder consistency.
3. Pour into glasses and serve immediately.

Time Frame: Preparation time: 5 minutes

Nutritional Information (per serving):
- Calories: 160 kcal
- Protein: 10g
- Carbohydrates: 25g
- Fat: 3g
- Fiber: 3g

10. Kiwi Strawberry Kale Smoothie:

Ingredients:
- 2 kiwi fruits, peeled and sliced
- 1/2 cup frozen strawberries
- 1 cup chopped kale leaves, stemmed
- 1/2 cup coconut water
- Juice of 1/2 lime
- Ice cubes (optional)

Instructions:

1. In a blender, combine the kiwi fruits, frozen strawberries, chopped kale leaves, coconut water, and lime juice.

2. Blend until smooth and creamy, adding ice cubes if desired for a colder consistency.

3. Pour into glasses and serve immediately.

Time Frame: Preparation time: 5 minutes

Nutritional Information (per serving):
- Calories: 130 kcal
- Protein: 3g
- Carbohydrates: 30g
- Fat: 1g
- Fiber: 6g

These recipes provide a delicious and nutritious way to incorporate fruits, vegetables, and other kidney-friendly ingredients into your diet, supporting overall health and well-being, especially for those managing stage 3 kidney disease. Enjoy!

Kidney-Friendly Brunch Ideas

1. Herb-Crusted Baked Salmon with Lemon-Dill Sauce:

Ingredients:
- 4 salmon fillets (6 oz each)
- 2 tablespoons olive oil
- 2 tablespoons fresh lemon juice
- 2 cloves garlic, minced
- 2 tablespoons chopped fresh dill
- 1/4 cup breadcrumbs
- Salt and pepper to taste

Lemon-Dill Sauce:

- 1/2 cup Greek yogurt
- 1 tablespoon fresh lemon juice
- 1 tablespoon chopped fresh dill
- Salt and pepper to taste

Instructions:

1. Preheat oven to 400°F (200°C). Line a baking sheet with parchment paper.
2. In a small bowl, mix together olive oil, lemon juice, garlic, and chopped dill.
3. Place salmon fillets on the prepared baking sheet. Brush the tops with the olive oil mixture.
4. In another bowl, mix breadcrumbs with salt and pepper. Sprinkle evenly over the salmon fillets, pressing lightly to adhere.
5. Bake for 12-15 minutes, or until the salmon is cooked through and flakes easily with a fork.
6. Meanwhile, prepare the lemon-dill sauce by mixing together Greek yogurt, lemon juice, chopped dill, salt, and pepper.
7. Serve the baked salmon hot with lemon-dill sauce on the side.

Time Frame: Prep Time: 10 minutes | Cook Time: 12-15 minutes | Total Time: 25 minutes

Nutritional Information (per serving):
- Calories: 350
- Protein: 35g
- Fat: 18g
- Carbohydrates: 10g
- Fiber: 1g

2. Mediterranean Chickpea Salad with Feta and Cucumber:

Ingredients:

- 2 cans chickpeas (15 oz each), drained and rinsed
- 1 cucumber, diced
- 1 cup cherry tomatoes, halved
- 1/2 cup crumbled feta cheese
- 1/4 cup chopped fresh parsley
- 1/4 cup chopped fresh mint
- 2 tablespoons extra virgin olive oil
- 2 tablespoons fresh lemon juice
- Salt and pepper to taste

Instructions:

1. In a large bowl, combine chickpeas, diced cucumber, cherry tomatoes, crumbled feta cheese, chopped parsley, and chopped mint.
2. In a small bowl, whisk together olive oil, lemon juice, salt, and pepper.
3. Pour the dressing over the salad and toss gently to coat.
4. Serve immediately or refrigerate until ready to serve.

Time Frame: Prep Time: 10 minutes | Total Time: 10 minutes

Nutritional Information (per serving):
- Calories: 220
- Protein: 9g
- Fat: 10g
- Carbohydrates: 26g
- Fiber: 6g

3. Whole Grain Pancakes with Blueberry Compote:

Ingredients:
- 1 cup whole wheat flour
- 1 tablespoon baking powder
- 1 tablespoon sugar

- 1/4 teaspoon salt
- 1 cup milk (or plant-based milk)
- 1 egg
- 2 tablespoons unsalted butter, melted
- 1 cup fresh or frozen blueberries

Blueberry Compote:
- 1 cup fresh or frozen blueberries
- 2 tablespoons maple syrup
- 1 tablespoon lemon juice

Instructions:

1. In a large bowl, whisk together whole wheat flour, baking powder, sugar, and salt.

2. In another bowl, whisk together milk, egg, and melted butter.

3. Pour the wet ingredients into the dry ingredients and stir until just combined. Fold in the blueberries.

4. Heat a lightly greased skillet or griddle over medium heat. Pour 1/4 cup of batter onto the skillet for each pancake.

5. Cook until bubbles form on the surface, then flip and cook until golden brown on the other side.

6. Meanwhile, prepare the blueberry compote by combining blueberries, maple syrup, and lemon juice in a small saucepan. Cook over medium heat, stirring occasionally, until the blueberries burst and the mixture thickens slightly.

7. Serve the pancakes hot with blueberry compote on top.

Time Frame: Prep Time: 10 minutes | Cook Time: 15 minutes | Total Time: 25 minutes

Nutritional Information (per serving, including blueberry compote):
- Calories: 270

- Protein: 7g
- Fat: 8g
- Carbohydrates: 45g
- Fiber: 5g

4. Veggie Egg White Frittata with Goat Cheese:

Ingredients:
- 8 egg whites
- 1/4 cup chopped red bell pepper
- 1/4 cup chopped green bell pepper
- 1/4 cup chopped onion
- 1/4 cup chopped spinach
- 1/4 cup crumbled goat cheese
- Salt and pepper to taste
- Cooking spray

Instructions:
1. Preheat oven to 350°F (175°C).
2. In a bowl, whisk together egg whites, chopped bell peppers, chopped onion, chopped spinach, salt, and pepper.
3. Lightly coat a skillet with cooking spray and heat over medium heat.
4. Pour the egg mixture into the skillet and cook for 3-4 minutes, or until the edges begin to set.
5. Sprinkle crumbled goat cheese evenly over the top of the frittata.
6. Transfer the skillet to the preheated oven and bake for 10-12 minutes, or until the frittata is set and lightly golden on top.
7. Remove from the oven and let cool slightly before slicing and serving.

Time Frame: Prep Time: 10 minutes | Cook Time: 15-20 minutes | Total Time: 25-30 minutes

Nutritional Information (per serving):
- Calories: 100
- Protein: 15g
- Fat: 2g
- Carbohydrates: 5g
- Fiber: 1g

5. Avocado and Tomato Bruschetta on Whole Grain Toast:

Ingredients:
- 2 ripe avocados, diced
- 1 cup cherry tomatoes, diced
- 2 tablespoons fresh basil, chopped
- 1 tablespoon balsamic vinegar
- 1 tablespoon extra virgin olive oil
- Salt and pepper to taste
- 4 slices whole grain bread, toasted

Instructions:
1. In a bowl, combine diced avocado, diced cherry tomatoes, chopped basil, balsamic vinegar, olive oil, salt, and pepper.
2. Mix gently until well combined.
3. Spoon the avocado and tomato mixture onto the toasted whole grain bread slices.
4. Serve immediately as a delicious and nutritious breakfast bruschetta.

Time Frame: Prep Time: 10 minutes | Total Time: 10 minutes

Nutritional Information (per serving):
- Calories: 200
- Protein: 5g
- Fat: 11g

- Carbohydrates: 24g
- Fiber: 6g

6. Turkey and Vegetable Breakfast Casserole:

Ingredients:
- 6 large eggs
- 1 cup milk (or plant-based milk)
- 1/2 teaspoon garlic powder
- 1/2 teaspoon onion powder
- Salt and pepper to taste
- 1 cup diced turkey sausage
- 1 cup diced bell peppers
- 1 cup diced zucchini
- 1 cup diced mushrooms
- 1 cup shredded cheddar cheese
- Cooking spray

Instructions:
1. Preheat oven to 350°F (175°C). Lightly coat a baking dish with cooking spray.
2. In a large bowl, whisk together eggs, milk, garlic powder, onion powder, salt, and pepper.
3. Stir in diced turkey sausage, diced bell peppers, diced zucchini, diced mushrooms, and shredded cheddar cheese.
4. Pour the egg mixture into the prepared baking dish.
5. Bake for 25-30 minutes, or until the casserole is set and golden brown on top.
6. Let cool slightly before slicing and serving.

Time Frame: Prep Time: 15 minutes | Cook Time: 25-30 minutes | Total Time: 40-45 minutes

Nutritional Information (per serving):
- Calories: 250
- Protein: 18g
- Fat: 15g
- Carbohydrates: 10g
- Fiber: 2g

7. Spinach and Mushroom Quiche with Whole Wheat Crust:

Ingredients:
- 1 whole wheat pie crust (store-bought or homemade)
- 6 large eggs
- 1 cup milk (or plant-based milk)
- 1 cup fresh spinach, chopped
- 1 cup sliced mushrooms
- 1/2 cup diced onion
- 1/2 cup shredded mozzarella cheese
- Salt and pepper to taste

Instructions:
1. Preheat oven to 375°F (190°C). Place the whole wheat pie crust in a pie dish.
2. In a bowl, whisk together eggs, milk, salt, and pepper.
3. Spread chopped spinach, sliced mushrooms, diced onion, and shredded mozzarella cheese evenly over the bottom of the pie crust.
4. Pour the egg mixture over the vegetables and cheese.
5. Bake for 35-40 minutes, or until the quiche is set and golden brown on top.
6. Let cool slightly before slicing and serving.

Time Frame: Prep Time: 15 minutes | Cook Time: 35-40 minutes | Total Time: 50-55 minutes

Nutritional Information (per serving):
- Calories: 280
- Protein: 14g
- Fat: 18g
- Carbohydrates: 17g
- Fiber: 3g

8. Smoked Turkey and Swiss Cheese Wraps with Whole Grain Tortillas:

Ingredients:
- 4 whole grain tortillas
- 8 slices smoked turkey breast
- 4 slices Swiss cheese
- 1 cup baby spinach leaves
- 1/2 cup sliced red bell pepper
- 1/4 cup sliced red onion
- 1/4 cup hummus

Instructions:
1. Lay out whole grain tortillas on a clean surface.
2. Spread hummus evenly over each tortilla.
3. Layer smoked turkey breast, Swiss cheese, baby spinach leaves, sliced red bell pepper, and sliced red onion evenly over each tortilla.
4. Roll up the tortillas tightly, tucking in the sides as you go.
5. Cut each wrap in half diagonally and serve immediately.

Time Frame: Prep Time: 10 minutes | Total Time: 10 minutes

Nutritional Information (per serving):
- Calories: 320
- Protein: 20g

- Fat: 15g
- Carbohydrates: 25g
- Fiber: 5g

9. Grilled Vegetable and Hummus Flatbread:

Ingredients:
- 2 whole grain flatbreads
- 1 cup hummus
- 1 cup sliced zucchini
- 1 cup sliced bell peppers
- 1 cup sliced red onion
- 1/2 cup crumbled feta cheese
- 2 tablespoons chopped fresh parsley
- 1 tablespoon olive oil
- Salt and pepper to taste

Instructions:
1. Preheat grill or grill pan to medium-high heat.
2. Brush sliced zucchini, bell peppers, and red onion with olive oil. Season with salt and pepper.
3. Grill vegetables for 3-4 minutes per side, or until tender and lightly charred.
4. Spread hummus evenly over each whole grain flatbread.
5. Top with grilled vegetables, crumbled feta cheese, and chopped fresh parsley.
6. Slice and serve immediately as a delicious and nutritious breakfast flatbread.

Time Frame: Prep Time: 10 minutes | Cook Time: 10 minutes | Total Time: 20 minutes

Nutritional Information (per serving):
- Calories: 350
- Protein: 12g
- Fat: 18g
- Carbohydrates: 35g
- Fiber: 8g

10. Banana Walnut Buckwheat Waffles with Maple Syrup:

Ingredients:
- 1 cup buckwheat flour
- 1 teaspoon baking powder
- 1/2 teaspoon baking soda
- 1/4 teaspoon salt
- 1 ripe banana, mashed
- 1 cup milk (or plant-based milk)
- 2 tablespoons maple syrup
- 1 egg
- 1/4 cup chopped walnuts

Instructions:
1. Preheat waffle iron according to manufacturer's instructions.
2. In a large bowl, whisk together buckwheat flour, baking powder, baking soda, and salt.
3. In another bowl, mix mashed banana, milk, maple syrup, and egg until well combined.
4. Pour the wet ingredients into the dry ingredients and stir until just combined. Fold in chopped walnuts.
5. Lightly coat the waffle iron with cooking spray. Pour batter onto the waffle iron and cook according to manufacturer's instructions, until golden brown and crispy.
6. Serve waffles hot with maple syrup drizzled on top.

Time Frame: Prep Time:

10 minutes | Cook Time: 10 minutes | Total Time: 20 minutes

Nutritional Information (per serving, including maple syrup):
- Calories: 300
- Protein: 9g
- Fat: 10g
- Carbohydrates: 45g
- Fiber: 6g

CHAPTER 3

SATISFYING SOUPS AND SALADS

Flavorful Soups for Every Season

1. Spicy Black Bean and Sweet Potato Soup:

Ingredients:
- 1 tablespoon olive oil
- 1 onion, diced
- 2 cloves garlic, minced
- 1 teaspoon ground cumin
- 1/2 teaspoon chili powder
- 1/4 teaspoon cayenne pepper (optional, adjust to taste)
- 2 sweet potatoes, peeled and diced
- 2 cans (15 oz each) black beans, drained and rinsed
- 4 cups vegetable broth
- Salt and pepper to taste
- Fresh cilantro, chopped (for garnish)
- Lime wedges (for serving)

Instructions:
1. In a large pot, heat olive oil over medium heat. Add onion and garlic, and cook until softened, about 5 minutes.
2. Add ground cumin, chili powder, and cayenne pepper (if using), and cook for an additional minute.
3. Stir in sweet potatoes, black beans, and vegetable broth. Bring to a boil.
4. Reduce heat and simmer until sweet potatoes are tender, about 20 minutes.
5. Use an immersion blender to partially puree the soup, leaving some chunks of sweet potato and black beans for texture. Alternatively, carefully transfer a

portion of the soup to a blender and blend until smooth, then return it to the pot.

6. Season with salt and pepper to taste.

7. Serve hot, garnished with chopped cilantro and lime wedges.

**Time frame: Prep Time: 15 minutes |Cook Time: 35 minutes |
Total Time: 50 minutes**

Nutritional Information (per serving):
- Calories: 240
- Total Fat: 3g
- Saturated Fat: 0g
- Cholesterol: 0mg
- Sodium: 680mg
- Total Carbohydrate: 47g
- Dietary Fiber: 13g
- Sugars: 6g
- Protein: 12g

2. Creamy Mushroom and Wild Rice Soup:

Ingredients:
- 1 tablespoon olive oil
- 1 onion, diced
- 2 cloves garlic, minced
- 8 oz mushrooms, sliced
- 1/2 cup wild rice
- 4 cups vegetable broth
- 1 cup unsweetened almond milk (or any unsweetened non-dairy milk)
- Salt and pepper to taste
- Fresh thyme, chopped (for garnish)

Instructions:

1. In a large pot, heat olive oil over medium heat. Add onion and garlic, and cook until softened, about 5 minutes.

2. Add mushrooms and cook until they release their liquid and start to brown, about 7-8 minutes.

3. Stir in wild rice and vegetable broth. Bring to a boil.

4. Reduce heat, cover, and simmer until rice is tender, about 45-50 minutes.

5. Stir in almond milk and heat through.

6. Season with salt and pepper to taste.

7. Serve hot, garnished with chopped fresh thyme.

Time Frame: Prep Time: 10 minutes | Cook Time: 60 minutes | Total Time: 70 minutes

Nutritional Information (per serving):

- Calories: 180
- Total Fat: 6g
- Saturated Fat: 1g
- Cholesterol: 0mg
- Sodium: 780mg
- Total Carbohydrate: 27g
- Dietary Fiber: 4g
- Sugars: 4g
- Protein: 5g

3. Thai Coconut Chicken Soup:

Ingredients:

- 1 tablespoon coconut oil
- 1 onion, diced
- 2 cloves garlic, minced
- 1 tablespoon grated fresh ginger

- 1 red bell pepper, thinly sliced
- 1 carrot, thinly sliced
- 4 cups chicken broth
- 1 can (14 oz) coconut milk
- 1 cup cooked chicken breast, shredded
- 2 tablespoons soy sauce (or tamari for gluten-free)
- 2 tablespoons lime juice
- 1 tablespoon fish sauce
- 1 teaspoon red curry paste
- Salt and pepper to taste
- Fresh cilantro, chopped (for garnish)
- Lime wedges (for serving)

Instructions:

1. In a large pot, heat coconut oil over medium heat. Add onion, garlic, and ginger, and cook until fragrant, about 2 minutes.
2. Add red bell pepper and carrot, and cook for an additional 3-4 minutes.
3. Stir in chicken broth, coconut milk, shredded chicken, soy sauce, lime juice, fish sauce, and red curry paste. Bring to a simmer.
4. Simmer for 10-15 minutes, until vegetables are tender and flavors are well combined.
5. Season with salt and pepper to taste.
6. Serve hot, garnished with chopped cilantro and lime wedges.

Time frame: Prep Time: 15 minutes | Cook Time: 25 minutes | Total Time: 40 minutes

Nutritional Information (per serving):
- Calories: 280
- Total Fat: 20g
- Saturated Fat: 16g
- Cholesterol: 25mg

- Sodium: 880mg
- Total Carbohydrate: 10g
- Dietary Fiber: 2g
- Sugars: 4g
- Protein: 15g

4. Moroccan Chickpea Stew:

Ingredients:
- 1 tablespoon olive oil
- 1 onion, diced
- 2 cloves garlic, minced
- 1 teaspoon ground cumin
- 1 teaspoon ground coriander
- 1/2 teaspoon ground cinnamon
- 1/2 teaspoon ground turmeric
- 1/4 teaspoon cayenne pepper (optional, adjust to taste)
- 2 cups vegetable broth
- 1 can (14 oz) diced tomatoes
- 1 can (15 oz) chickpeas, drained and rinsed
- 1 cup diced carrots
- 1 cup diced sweet potatoes
- 1/4 cup raisins
- Salt and pepper to taste
- Fresh cilantro, chopped (for garnish)
- Cooked couscous or quinoa (for serving)

Instructions:
1. In a large pot, heat olive oil over medium heat. Add onion and garlic, and cook until softened, about 5 minutes.
2. Add ground cumin, coriander, cinnamon, turmeric, and cayenne pepper (if using), and cook for an additional minute.

3. Stir in vegetable broth, diced tomatoes, chickpeas, carrots, sweet potatoes, and raisins. Bring to a boil.

4. Reduce heat and simmer, covered, for 20-25 minutes, until vegetables are tender.

5. Season with salt and pepper to taste.

6. Serve hot, garnished with chopped cilantro, and serve over cooked couscous or quinoa if desired.

Time Frame: Prep Time: 15 minutes | Cook Time: 30 minutes | Total Time: 45 minutes

Nutritional Information (per serving, without couscous or quinoa):
- Calories: 240
- Total Fat: 4g
- Saturated Fat: 0.5g
- Cholesterol: 0mg
- Sodium: 680mg
- Total Carbohydrate: 46g
- Dietary Fiber: 10g
- Sugars: 12g
- Protein: 9g

5. Italian Wedding Soup with Turkey Meatballs:

Ingredients:
- 1 tablespoon olive oil
- 1 onion, diced
- 2 carrots, diced
- 2 celery stalks, diced
- 2 cloves garlic, minced
- 8 cups chicken broth
- 1 cup small pasta (such as acini di pepe or orzo)

- 1 batch turkey meatballs (see below)
- 4 cups baby spinach
- Salt and pepper to taste
- Grated Parmesan cheese (for serving)

Turkey Meatballs:
- 1 lb ground turkey
- 1/4 cup breadcrumbs (gluten-free if necessary)
- 1/4 cup grated Parmesan cheese
- 1 egg
- 2 cloves garlic, minced
- 2 tablespoons chopped fresh parsley
- Salt and pepper to taste

Instructions:
1. In a large pot, heat olive oil over medium heat. Add onion, carrots, and celery. Cook until vegetables are softened, about 5 minutes.
2. Add garlic and cook for an additional minute.
3. Stir in chicken broth and bring to a simmer.
4. Meanwhile, prepare the turkey meatballs. In a mixing bowl, combine ground turkey, breadcrumbs, Parmesan cheese, egg, garlic, parsley, salt, and pepper. Shape into small meatballs.
5. Carefully drop meatballs into the simmering broth. Cook for 10-12 minutes, until meatballs are cooked through.
6. Stir in pasta and cook according to package instructions.
7. Add baby spinach and cook until wilted, about 2 minutes.
8. Season with salt and pepper to taste.
9. Serve hot, garnished with grated Parmesan cheese.

Time frame: Prep Time: 20 minutes
| Cook Time: 25 minutes
| Total Time: 45 minutes

Nutritional Information (per serving, without Parmesan cheese):
- Calories: 300
- Total Fat: 10g
- Saturated Fat: 2.5g
- Cholesterol: 80mg
- Sodium: 860mg
- Total Carbohydrate: 28g
- Dietary Fiber: 4g
- Sugars: 4g
- Protein: 24g

6. Garden Harvest Minestrone:

Ingredients:
- 2 tablespoons olive oil
- 1 onion, diced
- 2 carrots, diced
- 2 celery stalks, diced
- 2 cloves garlic, minced
- 1 zucchini, diced
- 1 yellow squash, diced
- 1 can (14 oz) diced tomatoes
- 6 cups vegetable broth
- 1 can (15 oz) kidney beans, drained and rinsed
- 1 cup green beans, trimmed and cut into 1-inch pieces
- 1 cup small pasta (such as ditalini or elbow)
- 1 teaspoon dried oregano
- 1 teaspoon dried basil
- Salt and pepper to taste
- Fresh parsley, chopped (for garnish)
- Grated Parmesan cheese (optional, for serving)

Instructions:

1. In a large pot, heat olive oil over medium heat. Add onion, carrots, and celery. Cook until vegetables are softened, about 5 minutes.

2. Add garlic and cook for an additional minute.

3. Stir in zucchini, yellow squash, diced tomatoes, vegetable broth, kidney beans, green beans, oregano, and basil. Bring to a boil.

4. Reduce heat and simmer for 20 minutes.

5. Stir in pasta and continue to simmer until pasta is cooked, about 10 minutes.

6. Season with salt and pepper to taste.

7. Serve hot, garnished with chopped parsley and grated Parmesan cheese if desired.

Time Frame: Prep Time: 15 minutes| Cook Time: 35 minutes | Total Time: 50 minutes

Nutritional Information (per serving, without Parmesan cheese):
- Calories: 210
- Total Fat: 4g
- Saturated Fat: 0.5g
- Cholesterol: 0mg
- Sodium: 680mg
- Total Carbohydrate: 35g
- Dietary Fiber: 7g
- Sugars: 6g
- Protein: 8g

7. Coconut Curry Lentil Soup:

Ingredients:
- 1 tablespoon coconut oil

- 1 onion, diced
- 2 carrots, diced
- 2 celery stalks, diced
- 3 cloves garlic, minced
- 1 tablespoon curry powder
- 1 teaspoon ground cumin
- 1 teaspoon ground coriander
- 1 cup dried brown lentils, rinsed and drained
- 1 can (14 oz) coconut milk
- 4 cups vegetable broth
- 1 cup diced tomatoes
- Salt and pepper to taste
- Fresh cilantro, chopped (for garnish)
- Lime wedges (for serving)

Instructions:

1. In a large pot, heat coconut oil over medium heat. Add onion, carrots, and celery. Cook until vegetables are softened, about 5 minutes.

2. Add garlic, curry powder, cumin, and coriander. Cook for an additional minute.

3. Stir in lentils, coconut milk, vegetable broth, and diced tomatoes. Bring to a boil.

4. Reduce heat and simmer, covered, for 25-30 minutes or until lentils are tender.

5. Season with salt and pepper to taste.

6. Serve hot, garnished with chopped cilantro and lime wedges.

Time frames: Prep Time: 10 minutes | Cook Time: 35 minutes | Total Time: 45 minutes

Nutritional Information (per serving):
- Calories: 280

- Total Fat: 15g
- Saturated Fat: 12g
- Cholesterol: 0mg
- Sodium: 780mg
- Total Carbohydrate: 30g
- Dietary Fiber: 11g
- Sugars: 5g
- Protein: 10g

8. Roasted Tomato Basil Bisque:

Ingredients:
- 2 lbs tomatoes, halved
- 4 cloves garlic, peeled
- 1 onion, quartered
- 2 tablespoons olive oil
- Salt and pepper to taste
- 4 cups vegetable broth
- 1 cup fresh basil leaves, packed
- 1/2 cup heavy cream
- Optional: Croutons and additional fresh basil leaves (for garnish)

Instructions:
1. Preheat oven to 400°F (200°C).
2. Place tomatoes, garlic, and onion on a baking sheet. Drizzle with olive oil and season with salt and pepper.
3. Roast in the preheated oven for 25-30 minutes, or until vegetables are caramelized.
4. Transfer roasted vegetables to a large pot. Add vegetable broth and fresh basil leaves.
5. Use an immersion blender to puree the soup until smooth. Alternatively, carefully transfer the soup in batches to a blender and blend until smooth.

6. Return the soup to the pot and stir in heavy cream. Heat over medium-low heat until warmed through.

7. Season with additional salt and pepper if needed.

8. Serve hot, garnished with croutons and fresh basil leaves if desired.

Time frame: Prep Time: 10 minutes | Cook Time: 35 minutes | Total Time: 45 minutes

Nutritional Information (per serving, without garnishes):
- Calories: 180
- Total Fat: 14g
- Saturated Fat: 6g
- Cholesterol: 25mg
- Sodium: 780mg
- Total Carbohydrate: 14g
- Dietary Fiber: 3g
- Sugars: 7g
- Protein: 3g

9. Lemon Chicken Orzo Soup:

Ingredients:
- 1 tablespoon olive oil
- 1 onion, diced
- 2 carrots, diced
- 2 celery stalks, diced
- 2 cloves garlic, minced
- 6 cups chicken broth
- 1 cup cooked chicken breast, shredded
- 1/2 cup uncooked orzo pasta
- 2 tablespoons lemon juice
- 2 teaspoons lemon zest

- Salt and pepper to taste
- Fresh parsley, chopped (for garnish)

Instructions:

1. In a large pot, heat olive oil over medium heat. Add onion, carrots, and celery. Cook until vegetables are softened, about 5 minutes.
2. Add garlic and cook for an additional minute.
3. Stir in chicken broth, shredded chicken, and orzo pasta. Bring to a boil.
4. Reduce heat and simmer until orzo is cooked, about 10 minutes.
5. Stir in lemon juice and lemon zest. Season with salt and pepper to taste.
6. Serve hot, garnished with chopped parsley.

Time frame: Prep Time: 10 minutes | Cook Time: 25 minutes | Total Time: 35 minutes

Nutritional Information (per serving):
- Calories: 190
- Total Fat: 4g
- Saturated Fat: 1g
- Cholesterol: 25mg
- Sodium: 780mg
- Total Carbohydrate: 20g
- Dietary Fiber: 2g
- Sugars: 3g
- Protein: 17g

10. Butternut Squash and Apple Soup:

Ingredients:
- 1 butternut squash, peeled, seeded, and cubed
- 2 apples, peeled, cored, and diced
- 1 onion, diced

- 2 cloves garlic, minced
- 4 cups vegetable broth
- 1 teaspoon ground cinnamon
- 1/2 teaspoon ground nutmeg
- Salt and pepper to taste
- Optional: Greek yogurt or sour cream (for serving)
- Optional: Toasted pumpkin seeds (for garnish)

Instructions:

1. In a large pot, combine butternut squash, apples, onion, garlic, vegetable broth, cinnamon, and nutmeg.

2. Bring to a boil, then reduce heat and simmer until squash and apples are tender, about 20 minutes.

3. Use an immersion blender to puree the soup until smooth. Alternatively, carefully transfer the soup in batches to a blender and blend until smooth.

4. Season with salt and pepper to taste.

5. Serve hot, topped with a dollop of Greek yogurt or sour cream and toasted pumpkin seeds if desired.

Time frame: Prep Time: 15 minutes Cook Time: 35 minutes | Total Time: 50 minutes

Nutritional Information (per serving, without toppings):
- Calories: 130
- Total Fat: 0.5g
- Saturated Fat: 0g
- Cholesterol: 0mg
- Sodium: 680mg
- Total Carbohydrate: 32g
- Dietary Fiber: 6g
- Sugars: 14g
- Protein: 2g

Creative Salad Combinations

1. Strawberry Spinach Salad with Goat Cheese and Almonds

Ingredients:
- 6 cups fresh baby spinach leaves
- 1 pint fresh strawberries, hulled and sliced
- 1/2 cup crumbled goat cheese
- 1/4 cup sliced almonds, toasted
- 2 tablespoons balsamic vinegar
- 1 tablespoon extra virgin olive oil
- 1 teaspoon honey
- Salt and pepper to taste

Instructions:
1. In a large bowl, combine the spinach, sliced strawberries, crumbled goat cheese, and toasted almonds.
2. In a small bowl, whisk together the balsamic vinegar, olive oil, honey, salt, and pepper to make the dressing.
3. Drizzle the dressing over the salad and toss gently to coat.
4. Serve immediately.

Time frame: Prep time: 15 minutes

Nutritional information (per serving):
- Calories: 180 kcal
- Protein: 7g
- Fat: 12g
- Carbohydrates: 15g
- Fiber: 4g

2. Mediterranean Quinoa Salad with Feta and Olives

Ingredients:
- 1 cup quinoa, rinsed
- 2 cups water or vegetable broth
- 1 cup cherry tomatoes, halved
- 1/2 cup cucumber, diced
- 1/4 cup Kalamata olives, sliced
- 1/4 cup crumbled feta cheese
- 2 tablespoons chopped fresh parsley
- 2 tablespoons lemon juice
- 2 tablespoons extra virgin olive oil
- Salt and pepper to taste

Instructions:
1. In a medium saucepan, bring the water or vegetable broth to a boil. Add the quinoa, reduce heat to low, cover, and simmer for 15-20 minutes, or until the quinoa is cooked and the liquid is absorbed.
2. In a large bowl, combine the cooked quinoa, cherry tomatoes, cucumber, olives, feta cheese, and parsley.
3. In a small bowl, whisk together the lemon juice, olive oil, salt, and pepper to make the dressing.
4. Drizzle the dressing over the salad and toss gently to coat.
5. Serve chilled or at room temperature.

Time frame: Prep time: 10 minutes, Cook time: 20 minutes

Nutritional information (per serving):
- Calories: 240 kcal
- Protein: 7g
- Fat: 12g
- Carbohydrates: 28g
- Fiber: 4g

3. Asian-Inspired Sesame Ginger Noodle Salad

Ingredients:
- 8 oz whole wheat spaghetti or soba noodles
- 2 cups shredded cabbage
- 1 red bell pepper, thinly sliced
- 1 carrot, julienned
- 1/4 cup green onions, sliced
- 1/4 cup cilantro, chopped
- 1/4 cup unsalted peanuts, chopped (optional)
- 2 tablespoons sesame seeds, toasted
- 1/4 cup soy sauce (low sodium)
- 2 tablespoons rice vinegar
- 1 tablespoon sesame oil
- 1 tablespoon honey
- 1 tablespoon fresh ginger, grated
- 1 clove garlic, minced
- Juice of 1 lime

Instructions:
1. Cook the noodles according to package instructions. Drain and rinse under cold water. Set aside.
2. In a large bowl, combine the cooked noodles, shredded cabbage, sliced bell pepper, julienned carrot, sliced green onions, chopped cilantro, chopped peanuts (if using), and toasted sesame seeds.
3. In a small bowl, whisk together the soy sauce, rice vinegar, sesame oil, honey, grated ginger, minced garlic, and lime juice to make the dressing.
4. Pour the dressing over the noodle salad and toss gently to coat.
5. Serve chilled or at room temperature.

Time frame: Prep time: 15 minutes, Cook time: 10 minutes

Nutritional information (per serving):
- Calories: 320 kcal
- Protein: 10g
- Fat: 10g
- Carbohydrates: 50g
- Fiber: 7g

4. Grilled Peach and Arugula Salad with Balsamic Glaze

Ingredients:
- 4 ripe peaches, halved and pitted
- 6 cups arugula
- 1/4 cup crumbled goat cheese
- 1/4 cup chopped walnuts, toasted
- Balsamic glaze for drizzling
- Salt and pepper to taste

Instructions:
1. Preheat grill to medium-high heat.
2. Place peach halves on the grill, cut side down, and grill for 3-4 minutes, until grill marks appear and peaches are slightly softened.
3. In a large bowl, combine arugula, grilled peaches, crumbled goat cheese, and toasted walnuts.
4. Drizzle balsamic glaze over the salad and season with salt and pepper.
5. Toss gently to combine and serve immediately.

Time frame: Prep time: 10 minutes, Cook time: 5 minutes

Nutritional information (per serving):
- Calories: 180 kcal
- Protein: 5g

- Fat: 9g
- Carbohydrates: 22g
- Fiber: 4g

5. Southwest BBQ Chicken Salad with Corn and Avocado

Ingredients:
- 2 boneless, skinless chicken breasts
- 1 tablespoon olive oil
- 1 teaspoon chili powder
- 1/2 teaspoon cumin
- 1/2 teaspoon paprika
- Salt and pepper to taste
- 6 cups mixed salad greens
- 1 cup canned black beans, rinsed and drained
- 1 cup corn kernels (fresh or canned)
- 1 avocado, diced
- 1/4 cup diced red onion
- 1/4 cup chopped fresh cilantro
- 1/4 cup BBQ sauce
- 2 tablespoons lime juice
- 2 tablespoons Greek yogurt (optional)

Instructions:
1. Preheat grill or grill pan over medium-high heat.
2. Brush chicken breasts with olive oil and season with chili powder, cumin, paprika, salt, and pepper.
3. Grill chicken for 6-8 minutes per side, or until cooked through. Remove from grill and let rest for 5 minutes before slicing.
4. In a large bowl, combine mixed salad greens, black beans, corn kernels, diced avocado, diced red onion, and chopped cilantro.

5. In a small bowl, whisk together BBQ sauce and lime juice to make the dressing.

6. Add sliced grilled chicken to the salad and drizzle with BBQ dressing. Optionally, add a dollop of Greek yogurt on top.

7. Toss gently to combine and serve immediately.

Time frame: Prep time: 15 minutes, Cook time: 15 minutes

Nutritional information (per serving):
- Calories: 350 kcal
- Protein: 25g
- Fat: 15g
- Carbohydrates: 30g
- Fiber: 8g

6. Citrus Shrimp and Mango Salad with Cilantro Lime Dressing

Ingredients:
- 1 lb large shrimp, peeled and deveined
- 2 tablespoons olive oil
- Salt and pepper to taste
- 6 cups mixed salad greens
- 1 mango, peeled, pitted, and diced
- 1/4 cup red onion, thinly sliced
- 1/4 cup chopped fresh cilantro
- 1/4 cup chopped roasted cashews (optional)
- 2 tablespoons lime juice
- 2 tablespoons orange juice
- 2 tablespoons honey
- 1 tablespoon extra virgin olive oil
- 1 teaspoon minced garlic
- Salt and pepper to taste

Instructions:

1. In a large skillet, heat olive oil over medium-high heat. Season shrimp with salt and pepper, then add to the skillet.

2. Cook shrimp for 2-3 minutes per side, or until pink and opaque. Remove from heat and set aside.

3. In a large bowl, combine mixed salad greens, diced mango, sliced red onion, chopped cilantro, and roasted cashews (if using).

4. In a small bowl, whisk together lime juice, orange juice, honey, olive oil, minced garlic, salt, and pepper to make the dressing.

5. Add cooked shrimp to the salad and drizzle with cilantro lime dressing.

6. Toss gently to combine and serve immediately.

Time frame: Prep time: 15 minutes, Cook time: 5 minutes

Nutritional information (per serving):

- Calories: 280 kcal
- Protein: 20g
- Fat: 14g
- Carbohydrates: 20g
- Fiber: 3g

7. Greek Orzo Pasta Salad with Cherry Tomatoes and Cucumber

Ingredients:

- 1 cup uncooked orzo pasta
- 1 cup cherry tomatoes, halved
- 1 cucumber, diced
- 1/4 cup sliced Kalamata olives
- 1/4 cup crumbled feta cheese
- 2 tablespoons chopped fresh parsley
- 2 tablespoons lemon juice

- 2 tablespoons extra virgin olive oil
- 1 teaspoon dried oregano
- Salt and pepper to taste

Instructions:

1. Cook orzo pasta according to package instructions. Drain and rinse under cold water.

2. In a large bowl, combine cooked orzo pasta, cherry tomatoes, diced cucumber, sliced Kalamata olives, crumbled feta cheese, and chopped fresh parsley.

3. In a small bowl, whisk together lemon juice, olive oil, dried oregano, salt, and pepper to make the dressing.

4. Pour the dressing over the pasta salad and toss gently to coat.

5. Serve chilled or at room temperature.

Time frame: Prep time: 10 minutes, Cook time: 10 minutes

Nutritional information (per serving):
- Calories: 250 kcal
- Protein: 7g
- Fat: 8g
- Carbohydrates: 37g
- Fiber: 3g

8. Roasted Beet and Goat Cheese Salad with Honey Dijon Dressing

Ingredients:
- 4 medium-sized beets, trimmed and peeled
- 4 cups mixed salad greens
- 1/4 cup crumbled goat cheese
- 1/4 cup chopped walnuts, toasted
- 2 tablespoons balsamic vinegar

- 1 tablespoon extra virgin olive oil
- 1 teaspoon honey
- 1 teaspoon Dijon mustard
- Salt and pepper to taste

Instructions:
1. Preheat oven to 400°F (200°C).
2. Cut the beets into bite-sized cubes and place them on a baking sheet lined with parchment paper.
3. Drizzle with olive oil, season with salt and pepper, and toss to coat.
4. Roast in the preheated oven for 25-30 minutes or until the beets are tender and caramelized.
5. In a small bowl, whisk together balsamic vinegar, olive oil, honey, Dijon mustard, salt, and pepper to make the dressing.
6. In a large bowl, combine mixed salad greens, roasted beets, crumbled goat cheese, and toasted walnuts.
7. Drizzle the dressing over the salad and toss gently to coat.
8. Serve immediately.

Time frame: Prep time: 15 minutes, Cook time: 25-30 minutes

Nutritional information (per serving):
- Calories: 220 kcal
- Protein: 7g
- Fat: 14g
- Carbohydrates: 20g
- Fiber: 5g

9. Caprese Salad Skewers with Basil Pesto Drizzle

Ingredients:
- 1 pint cherry tomatoes

- 8 oz fresh mozzarella cheese, cubed
- Fresh basil leaves
- Balsamic glaze, for drizzling
- Wooden skewers

Instructions:

1. Thread a cherry tomato, a basil leaf, and a cube of mozzarella cheese onto each wooden skewer.
2. Arrange the skewers on a serving platter.
3. Drizzle with balsamic glaze.
4. Serve immediately.

Time frame: Prep time: 10 minutes

Nutritional information (per serving):
- Calories: 80 kcal
- Protein: 5g
- Fat: 5g
- Carbohydrates: 3g
- Fiber: 1g

10. Harvest Farro Salad with Roasted Vegetables and Maple Dijon Dressing

Ingredients:
- 1 cup farro, rinsed
- 2 cups vegetable broth
- 1 cup Brussels sprouts, halved
- 1 cup butternut squash, diced
- 1/2 cup dried cranberries
- 1/4 cup chopped pecans, toasted
- 2 tablespoons maple syrup

- 1 tablespoon Dijon mustard
- 1 tablespoon apple cider vinegar
- 2 tablespoons extra virgin olive oil
- Salt and pepper to taste

Instructions:
1. In a medium saucepan, bring vegetable broth to a boil. Add farro, reduce heat to low, cover, and simmer for 20-25 minutes or until farro is tender and liquid is absorbed. Remove from heat and let cool.
2. Preheat oven to 400°F (200°C).
3. Place Brussels sprouts and butternut squash on a baking sheet lined with parchment paper. Drizzle with olive oil, maple syrup, salt, and pepper, and toss to coat.
4. Roast in the preheated oven for 20-25 minutes or until vegetables are tender and caramelized.
5. In a small bowl, whisk together Dijon mustard, apple cider vinegar, olive oil, salt, and pepper to make the dressing.
6. In a large bowl, combine cooked farro, roasted vegetables, dried cranberries, and toasted pecans.
7. Drizzle the dressing over the salad and toss gently to coat.
8. Serve chilled or at room temperature.

Time frame: Prep time: 20 minutes, Cook time: 25-30 minutes

Nutritional information (per serving):
- Calories: 280 kcal
- Protein: 5g
- Fat: 8g
- Carbohydrates: 50g
- Fiber: 8g

Enjoy preparing these delicious and nutritious salads!

Dressings and Vinaigrettes

1. Classic Balsamic Vinaigrette:

Ingredients:
- 1/4 cup balsamic vinegar
- 1 tablespoon Dijon mustard
- 1 clove garlic, minced
- 1/2 cup extra virgin olive oil
- Salt and pepper to taste

Instructions:
1. In a small bowl, whisk together balsamic vinegar, Dijon mustard, and minced garlic.
2. Slowly drizzle in the olive oil while whisking continuously until the dressing is emulsified.
3. Season with salt and pepper to taste.
4. Store in an airtight container in the refrigerator for up to one week.

Preparation Time: 5 minutes
Yield: About 3/4 cup
Nutritional Information (per serving - 2 tablespoons):
- Calories: 120
- Total Fat: 14g
- Saturated Fat: 2g
- Sodium: 50mg
- Total Carbohydrates: 1g
- Sugars: 0g
- Protein: 0g

2. Creamy Avocado Lime Dressing:

Ingredients:
- 1 ripe avocado, peeled and pitted
- Juice of 2 limes
- 1/4 cup plain Greek yogurt
- 2 tablespoons olive oil
- 1 clove garlic, minced
- Salt and pepper to taste

Instructions:
1. In a blender or food processor, combine the avocado, lime juice, Greek yogurt, olive oil, and minced garlic.
2. Blend until smooth and creamy.
3. Season with salt and pepper to taste.
4. Transfer to an airtight container and refrigerate until ready to use.

Preparation Time: 5 minutes
Yield: About 1 cup
Nutritional Information (per serving - 2 tablespoons):
- Calories: 60
- Total Fat: 5g
- Saturated Fat: 1g
- Sodium: 15mg
- Total Carbohydrates: 3g
- Sugars: 0g
- Protein: 1g

3. Honey Mustard Dijon Dressing:

Ingredients:
- 1/4 cup Dijon mustard
- 2 tablespoons honey
- 2 tablespoons apple cider vinegar

- 1/4 cup olive oil
- Salt and pepper to taste

Instructions:

1. In a small bowl, whisk together Dijon mustard, honey, and apple cider vinegar until well combined.
2. Slowly drizzle in the olive oil while whisking continuously until the dressing is emulsified.
3. Season with salt and pepper to taste.
4. Store in an airtight container in the refrigerator for up to one week.

Preparation Time: 5 minutes
Yield: About 3/4 cup
Nutritional Information (per serving - 2 tablespoons):
- Calories: 120
- Total Fat: 11g
- Saturated Fat: 1.5g
- Sodium: 150mg
- Total Carbohydrates: 6g
- Sugars: 5g
- Protein: 0g

4. Greek Yogurt Ranch Dressing:

Ingredients:
- 1/2 cup plain Greek yogurt
- 1/4 cup buttermilk
- 1 tablespoon chopped fresh dill
- 1 tablespoon chopped fresh chives
- 1 clove garlic, minced
- Juice of 1/2 lemon
- Salt and pepper to taste

Instructions:

1. In a small bowl, whisk together Greek yogurt and buttermilk until smooth.
2. Stir in chopped dill, chives, minced garlic, and lemon juice until well combined.
3. Season with salt and pepper to taste.
4. Store in an airtight container in the refrigerator for up to one week.

Preparation Time: 5 minutes
Yield: About 3/4 cup
Nutritional Information (per serving - 2 tablespoons):
- Calories: 30
- Total Fat: 1g
- Saturated Fat: 0.5g
- Sodium: 50mg
- Total Carbohydrates: 2g
- Sugars: 1g
- Protein: 3g

5. Raspberry Walnut Vinaigrette:

Ingredients:
- 1/4 cup raspberry vinegar
- 1/4 cup extra virgin olive oil
- 1 tablespoon honey
- 2 tablespoons chopped walnuts
- Salt and pepper to taste

Instructions:

1. In a small bowl, whisk together raspberry vinegar, olive oil, and honey until well combined.
2. Stir in chopped walnuts.

3. Season with salt and pepper to taste.

4. Store in an airtight container in the refrigerator for up to one week.

Preparation Time: 5 minutes
Yield: About 1/2 cup
Nutritional Information (per serving - 2 tablespoons):
- Calories: 120
- Total Fat: 12g
- Saturated Fat: 1.5g
- Sodium: 0mg
- Total Carbohydrates: 3g
- Sugars: 3g
- Protein: 0g

6. Tahini Lemon Herb Dressing:

Ingredients:
- 1/4 cup tahini
- Juice of 1 lemon
- 2 tablespoons water
- 1 clove garlic, minced
- 1 tablespoon chopped fresh parsley
- 1 tablespoon chopped fresh cilantro
- Salt and pepper to taste

Instructions:
1. In a small bowl, whisk together tahini, lemon juice, and water until smooth.
2. Stir in minced garlic, chopped parsley, and chopped cilantro until well combined.
3. Season with salt and pepper to taste.
4. Store in an airtight container in the refrigerator for up to one week.

Preparation Time: 5 minutes
Yield: About 1/2 cup
Nutritional Information (per serving - 2 tablespoons):
- Calories: 80
- Total Fat: 7g
- Saturated Fat: 1g
- Sodium: 40mg
- Total Carbohydrates: 4g
- Sugars: 1g
- Protein: 2g

7. Orange Maple Dijon Vinaigrette:

Ingredients:
- 1/4 cup orange juice
- 2 tablespoons apple cider vinegar
- 1 tablespoon maple syrup
- 1 tablespoon Dijon mustard
- 1/4 cup olive oil
- Salt and pepper to taste

Instructions:
1. In a small bowl, whisk together orange juice, apple cider vinegar, maple syrup, and Dijon mustard until well combined.
2. Slowly drizzle in the olive oil while whisking continuously until the dressing is emulsified.
3. Season with salt and pepper to taste.
4. Store in an airtight container in the refrigerator for up to one week.

Preparation Time: 5 minutes
Yield: About 3/4 cup

Nutritional Information (per serving - 2 tablespoons):
- Calories: 80
- Total Fat: 7g
- Saturated Fat: 1g
- Sodium: 80mg
- Total Carbohydrates: 4g
- Sugars: 3g
- Protein: 0g

8. Asian Sesame Ginger Dressing:

Ingredients:
- 1/4 cup rice vinegar
- 2 tablespoons soy sauce (low-sodium preferred)
- 1 tablespoon sesame oil
- 1 tablespoon honey
- 1 teaspoon grated fresh ginger
- 1 clove garlic, minced
- 2 tablespoons olive oil
- Sesame seeds for garnish (optional)

Instructions:
1. In a small bowl, whisk together rice vinegar, soy sauce, sesame oil, honey, grated ginger, and minced garlic until well combined.
2. Slowly drizzle in the olive oil while whisking continuously until the dressing is emulsified.
3. Garnish with sesame seeds if desired.
4. Store in an airtight container in the refrigerator for up to one week.

Preparation Time: 5 minutes
Yield: About 1/2 cup
Nutritional Information (per serving - 2 tablespoons):

- Calories: 60
- Total Fat: 5g
- Saturated Fat: 0.5g
- Sodium: 150mg
- Total Carbohydrates: 4g
- Sugars: 3g
- Protein: 0g

9. Cilantro Lime Vinaigrette:

Ingredients:
- 1/4 cup lime juice
- 1/4 cup extra virgin olive oil
- 1/4 cup chopped fresh cilantro
- 1 clove garlic, minced
- 1 teaspoon honey
- Salt and pepper to taste

Instructions:
1. In a small bowl, whisk together lime juice, olive oil, chopped cilantro, minced garlic, and honey until well combined.
2. Season with salt and pepper to taste.
3. Store in an airtight container in the refrigerator for up to one week.

Preparation Time: 5 minutes
Yield: About 3/4 cup
Nutritional Information (per serving - 2 tablespoons):
- Calories: 120
- Total Fat: 14g
- Saturated Fat: 2g
- Sodium: 0mg
- Total Carbohydrates: 2g

- Sugars: 1g
- Protein: 0g

10. Apple Cider Vinaigrette with Shallots:

Ingredients:
- 1/4 cup apple cider vinegar
- 1/4 cup extra virgin olive oil
- 1 shallot, finely minced
- 1 teaspoon Dijon mustard
- 1 teaspoon honey
- Salt and pepper to taste

Instructions:
1. In a small bowl, whisk together apple cider vinegar, olive oil, minced shallot, Dijon mustard, and honey until well combined.
2. Season with salt and pepper to taste.
3. Store in an airtight container in the refrigerator for up to one week.

Preparation Time: 5 minutes
Yield: About 3/4 cup
Nutritional Information (per serving - 2 tablespoons):
- Calories: 120
- Total Fat: 14g
- Saturated Fat: 2g
- Sodium: 30mg
- Total Carbohydrates: 2g
- Sugars: 1g
- Protein: 0g

Chapter 4

Hearty Main Dishes

Protein-Packed Poultry and Fish

1. Lemon Herb Grilled Chicken Breast:

Preparation Time: 35 minutes (including marination)
Cooking Time: 12-16 minutes
Total Time: 47-51 minutes

Ingredients:
- 4 boneless, skinless chicken breasts
- 2 tablespoons olive oil
- 2 tablespoons fresh lemon juice
- 2 cloves garlic, minced
- 1 teaspoon dried oregano
- 1 teaspoon dried thyme
- Salt and pepper to taste
- Lemon wedges for garnish

Instructions:
1. In a small bowl, whisk together olive oil, lemon juice, minced garlic, dried oregano, dried thyme, salt, and pepper to create a marinade.
2. Place chicken breasts in a shallow dish or resealable plastic bag. Pour marinade over chicken, ensuring all pieces are evenly coated. Marinate in the refrigerator for at least 30 minutes, or up to 4 hours for maximum flavor.
3. Preheat grill to medium-high heat. Remove chicken from marinade and discard excess marinade.

4. Grill chicken breasts for 6-8 minutes per side, or until internal temperature reaches 165°F (75°C) and juices run clear.

5. Remove from grill and let rest for 5 minutes before serving. Garnish with lemon wedges and serve hot.

Nutritional Information (per serving):
- Calories: 220
- Protein: 30g
- Fat: 9g
- Carbohydrates: 2g
- Fiber: 0.5g

2. Garlic Butter Baked Salmon:

Preparation Time: 10 minutes
Cooking Time: 12-15 minutes
Total Time: 22-25 minutes

Ingredients:
- 4 salmon fillets (6 ounces each)
- 4 tablespoons unsalted butter, melted
- 4 cloves garlic, minced
- 2 tablespoons fresh lemon juice
- 1 tablespoon chopped fresh parsley
- Salt and pepper to taste
- Lemon slices for garnish

Instructions:
1. Preheat oven to 375°F (190°C). Line a baking sheet with parchment paper or lightly grease with cooking spray.

2. Place salmon fillets on the prepared baking sheet. In a small bowl, mix together melted butter, minced garlic, lemon juice, chopped parsley, salt, and pepper.

3. Spoon the garlic butter mixture evenly over the salmon fillets.

4. Bake in preheated oven for 12-15 minutes, or until salmon flakes easily with a fork and reaches an internal temperature of 145°F (63°C).

5. Remove from oven and let rest for a few minutes before serving. Garnish with lemon slices and serve hot.

Nutritional Information (per serving):
- Calories: 380
- Protein: 34g
- Fat: 24g
- Carbohydrates: 1g
- Fiber: 0.5g

3. Rosemary Roasted Turkey Breast:

Preparation Time: 10 minutes
Cooking Time: 60-75 minutes
Total Time: 70-85 minutes

Ingredients:
- 1 turkey breast (about 2-3 pounds)
- 2 tablespoons olive oil
- 2 cloves garlic, minced
- 1 tablespoon chopped fresh rosemary
- 1 teaspoon dried thyme
- Salt and pepper to taste
- 1 lemon, sliced (optional)
- Fresh rosemary sprigs for garnish (optional)

Instructions:

1. Preheat oven to 375°F (190°C).

2. In a small bowl, combine olive oil, minced garlic, chopped fresh rosemary, dried thyme, salt, and pepper to create a marinade.

3. Place turkey breast in a roasting pan or baking dish. Rub the marinade all over the turkey breast, ensuring it is evenly coated.

4. If desired, place lemon slices on top of the turkey breast for additional flavor.

5. Roast in the preheated oven for 60-75 minutes, or until turkey reaches an internal temperature of 165°F (75°C) and juices run clear.

6. Remove from oven and let rest for 10 minutes before slicing. Garnish with fresh rosemary sprigs if desired.

Nutritional Information (per serving):
- Calories: 240
- Protein: 40g
- Fat: 7g
- Carbohydrates: 0g
- Fiber: 0g

4. Spicy Cajun Blackened Tilapia:

Preparation Time: 5 minutes
Cooking Time: 6-8 minutes
Total Time: 11-13 minutes

Ingredients:
- 4 tilapia fillets (6 ounces each)
- 2 tablespoons olive oil
- 2 teaspoons Cajun seasoning
- 1 teaspoon paprika
- 1/2 teaspoon garlic powder

- 1/2 teaspoon onion powder
- 1/4 teaspoon cayenne pepper (adjust to taste)
- Salt and pepper to taste
- Lemon wedges for garnish

Instructions:

1. In a small bowl, mix together Cajun seasoning, paprika, garlic powder, onion powder, cayenne pepper, salt, and pepper to create a spice rub.

2. Pat tilapia fillets dry with paper towels. Rub both sides of each fillet with olive oil, then generously sprinkle with the spice rub, pressing gently to adhere.

3. Heat a large skillet or grill pan over medium-high heat. Once hot, add tilapia fillets to the pan (you may need to work in batches depending on the size of your pan).

4. Cook tilapia for 3-4 minutes per side, or until fish is blackened and flakes easily with a fork.

5. Remove from heat and serve hot with lemon wedges for garnish.

Nutritional Information (per serving):
- Calories: 200
- Protein: 30g
- Fat: 8g
- Carbohydrates: 1g
- Fiber: 0g

5. Mediterranean Chicken Skewers with Tzatziki Sauce:

Preparation Time: 40 minutes (including marination)
Cooking Time: 10-12 minutes
Total Time: 50-52 minutes

Ingredients:

- 1 pound boneless, skinless chicken breasts, cut into 1-inch cubes
- 2 tablespoons olive oil
- 2 cloves garlic, minced
- 1 teaspoon dried oregano
- 1 teaspoon dried thyme
- 1 teaspoon dried rosemary
- Salt and pepper to taste
- Lemon wedges for garnish
- Wooden skewers, soaked in water for 30 minutes

For Tzatziki Sauce:
- 1 cup Greek yogurt
- 1/2 cucumber, grated and squeezed to remove excess moisture
- 2 cloves garlic, minced
- 1 tablespoon lemon juice
- 1 tablespoon chopped fresh dill
- Salt and pepper to taste

Instructions:

1. In a medium bowl, combine olive oil, minced garlic, dried oregano, dried thyme, dried rosemary, salt, and pepper. Add chicken cubes to the bowl and toss to coat evenly. Cover and marinate in the refrigerator for at least 30 minutes.

2. While the chicken is marinating, prepare the tzatziki sauce. In a small bowl, mix together Greek yogurt, grated cucumber, minced garlic, lemon juice, chopped fresh dill, salt, and pepper. Refrigerate until ready to serve.

3. Preheat grill to medium-high heat. Thread marinated chicken cubes onto soaked wooden skewers.

4. Grill chicken skewers for 5-7 minutes per side, or until chicken is cooked through and lightly charred.

5. Serve hot with tzatziki sauce on the side for dipping.

Nutritional Information (per serving, chicken skewers only):
- Calories: 250
- Protein: 30g
- Fat: 12g
- Carbohydrates: 2g
- Fiber: 0.5g

6. Honey Mustard Glazed Turkey Meatballs:

Preparation Time: 15 minutes
Cooking Time: 20-25 minutes
Total Time: 35-40 minutes

Ingredients:
- 1 pound ground turkey
- 1/4 cup breadcrumbs
- 1 egg
- 2 tablespoons honey
- 2 tablespoons Dijon mustard
- 1 tablespoon olive oil
- 1 tablespoon apple cider vinegar
- Salt and pepper to taste
- Chopped fresh parsley for garnish (optional)

Instructions:
1. Preheat oven to 400°F (200°C). Line a baking sheet with parchment paper.
2. In a large bowl, combine ground turkey, breadcrumbs, egg, salt, and pepper. Mix until well combined.
3. Shape the turkey mixture into meatballs, about 1 inch in diameter, and place them on the prepared baking sheet.
4. In a small bowl, whisk together honey, Dijon mustard, olive oil, and apple cider vinegar to make the glaze.

5. Brush the honey mustard glaze over the meatballs, coating them evenly.

6. Bake in the preheated oven for 20-25 minutes, or until meatballs are cooked through and golden brown.

7. Remove from oven and let cool for a few minutes before serving. Garnish with chopped fresh parsley if desired.

Nutritional Information (per serving, about 4 meatballs):
- Calories: 280
- Protein: 22g
- Fat: 16g
- Carbohydrates: 12g
- Fiber: 1g

7. Sesame Ginger Glazed Mahi-Mahi:

Preparation Time: 10 minutes
Cooking Time: 10-12 minutes
Total Time: 20-22 minutes

Ingredients:
- 4 mahi-mahi fillets (6 ounces each)
- 2 tablespoons soy sauce
- 1 tablespoon honey
- 1 tablespoon rice vinegar
- 1 tablespoon sesame oil
- 1 tablespoon grated fresh ginger
- 2 cloves garlic, minced
- 1 tablespoon sesame seeds
- Salt and pepper to taste
- Sliced green onions for garnish

Instructions:

1. In a small bowl, whisk together soy sauce, honey, rice vinegar, sesame oil, grated ginger, minced garlic, sesame seeds, salt, and pepper to make the glaze.

2. Pat mahi-mahi fillets dry with paper towels. Place them in a shallow dish and pour the glaze over the fillets, ensuring they are evenly coated. Marinate for 10-15 minutes.

3. Preheat grill or grill pan to medium-high heat. Remove mahi-mahi fillets from the marinade and discard excess marinade.

4. Grill mahi-mahi fillets for 4-6 minutes per side, or until fish is cooked through and flakes easily with a fork.

5. Remove from grill and let rest for a few minutes before serving. Garnish with sliced green onions and serve hot.

Nutritional Information (per serving):
- Calories: 280
- Protein: 32g
- Fat: 10g
- Carbohydrates: 10g
- Fiber: 1g

8. Herb-Crusted Baked Cod Fillets:

Preparation Time: 10 minutes
Cooking Time: 15-20 minutes
Total Time: 25-30 minutes

Ingredients:
- 4 cod fillets (6 ounces each)
- 1/4 cup breadcrumbs
- 1 tablespoon grated Parmesan cheese
- 1 teaspoon dried parsley
- 1 teaspoon dried thyme

- 1 teaspoon dried oregano
- 1/2 teaspoon garlic powder
- 1/2 teaspoon onion powder
- 2 tablespoons olive oil
- Lemon wedges for garnish
- Fresh parsley for garnish

Instructions:
1. Preheat oven to 400°F (200°C). Line a baking sheet with parchment paper.
2. In a small bowl, mix together breadcrumbs, Parmesan cheese, dried parsley, dried thyme, dried oregano, garlic powder, onion powder, salt, and pepper.
3. Pat cod fillets dry with paper towels. Brush each fillet with olive oil, then press the breadcrumb mixture onto the top of each fillet to create a crust.
4. Place cod fillets on the prepared baking sheet. Bake in the preheated oven for 15-20 minutes, or until fish is opaque and flakes easily with a fork.
5. Remove from oven and let cool for a few minutes before serving. Garnish with lemon wedges and fresh parsley before serving.

Nutritional Information (per serving):
- Calories: 220
- Protein: 30g
- Fat: 9g
- Carbohydrates: 4g
- Fiber: 0.5g

9. Teriyaki Chicken Stir-Fry:

Preparation Time: 15 minutes
Cooking Time: 15 minutes
Total Time: 30 minutes

Ingredients:
- 1 pound boneless, skinless chicken breasts, thinly sliced
- 2 tablespoons soy sauce
- 2 tablespoons honey
- 1 tablespoon rice vinegar
- 1 tablespoon sesame oil
- 2 cloves garlic, minced
- 1 teaspoon grated fresh ginger
- 2 cups mixed vegetables (bell peppers, broccoli, carrots, snap peas, etc.)
- 2 tablespoons vegetable oil
- Cooked rice or noodles for serving
- Sesame seeds for garnish
- Sliced green onions for garnish

Instructions:

1. In a small bowl, whisk together soy sauce, honey, rice vinegar, sesame oil, minced garlic, and grated ginger to make the teriyaki sauce. Set aside.

2. Heat vegetable oil in a large skillet or wok over medium-high heat. Add sliced chicken breasts and stir-fry for 4-5 minutes, or until chicken is cooked through.

3. Add mixed vegetables to the skillet and continue to stir-fry for another 4-5 minutes, or until vegetables are tender-crisp.

4. Pour the teriyaki sauce over the chicken and vegetables. Stir well to coat everything evenly with the sauce.

5. Cook for an additional 2-3 minutes, or until the sauce has thickened slightly.

6. Serve hot over cooked rice or noodles. Garnish with sesame seeds and sliced green onions before serving.

Nutritional Information (per serving):
- Calories: 320
- Protein: 25g

- Fat: 12g
- Carbohydrates: 25g
- Fiber: 4g

10. Coconut Lime Grilled Shrimp Skewers:

Preparation Time: 20 minutes (including marination)
Cooking Time: 6-8 minutes
Total Time: 26-28 minutes

Ingredients:
- 1 pound large shrimp, peeled and deveined
- 1/4 cup coconut milk
- Zest and juice of 1 lime
- 2 cloves garlic, minced
- 1 tablespoon soy sauce
- 1 tablespoon honey
- 1 tablespoon chopped fresh cilantro
- 1 teaspoon grated fresh ginger
- Salt and pepper to taste
- Wooden skewers, soaked in water for 30 minutes

Instructions:
1. In a shallow dish, combine coconut milk, lime zest, lime juice, minced garlic, soy sauce, honey, chopped cilantro, grated ginger, salt, and pepper. Add shrimp to the dish and toss to coat evenly. Marinate in the refrigerator for 15-20 minutes.
2. Preheat grill to medium-high heat. Thread marinated shrimp onto soaked wooden skewers.
3. Grill shrimp skewers for 2-3 minutes per side, or until shrimp are pink and opaque.
4. Remove from grill and let cool for a few minutes before serving.

Nutritional Information (per serving):
- Calories: 180
- Protein: 24g
- Fat: 6g
- Carbohydrates: 6g
- Fiber: 0.5g

Vegetarian Delights for Seniors

1. Quinoa Stuffed Bell Peppers:

Ingredients:
- 4 large bell peppers (any color)
- 1 cup quinoa, rinsed
- 2 cups vegetable broth
- 1 can (15 oz) black beans, drained and rinsed
- 1 cup corn kernels (fresh, canned, or frozen)
- 1 cup diced tomatoes
- 1 teaspoon chili powder
- 1 teaspoon cumin
- Salt and pepper, to taste
- 1 cup shredded cheese (optional)

Instructions:
1. Preheat the oven to 375°F (190°C). Grease a baking dish with cooking spray.
2. Cut the tops off the bell peppers and remove the seeds and membranes. Place the peppers upright in the prepared baking dish.
3. In a medium saucepan, combine the quinoa and vegetable broth. Bring to a boil, then reduce the heat to low, cover, and simmer for 15 minutes, or until the quinoa is cooked and the liquid is absorbed.

4. In a large mixing bowl, combine the cooked quinoa, black beans, corn, diced tomatoes, chili powder, cumin, salt, and pepper. Mix well to combine.

5. Spoon the quinoa mixture into the hollowed-out bell peppers until they are filled to the top. If using cheese, sprinkle it over the top of each stuffed pepper.

6. Cover the baking dish with aluminum foil and bake in the preheated oven for 25-30 minutes, or until the peppers are tender.

7. Remove the foil and bake for an additional 5 minutes, or until the cheese is melted and bubbly.

8. Serve the quinoa stuffed bell peppers hot, garnished with fresh cilantro or chopped green onions if desired.

Time Frame: Prep Time: 15 minutes, Cook Time: 45-50 minutes, Total Time: 60-65 minutes

Nutritional Information (per serving, without cheese):
- Calories: 250 kcal
- Total Fat: 2.5 g
- Saturated Fat: 0.5 g
- Cholesterol: 0 mg
- Sodium: 350 mg
- Total Carbohydrates: 48 g
- Dietary Fiber: 9 g
- Sugars: 7 g
- Protein: 10 g

2. Lentil and Vegetable Shepherd's Pie:

Ingredients:
- 2 cups cooked lentils
- 2 tablespoons olive oil
- 1 onion, diced

- 2 carrots, diced
- 2 celery stalks, diced
- 2 cloves garlic, minced
- 1 cup frozen peas
- 1 cup corn kernels (fresh, canned, or frozen)
- 2 tablespoons tomato paste
- 1 cup vegetable broth
- 1 tablespoon Worcestershire sauce (optional)
- Salt and pepper, to taste
- 4 cups mashed potatoes (prepared)

Instructions:

1. Preheat the oven to 375°F (190°C). Grease a baking dish with cooking spray.

2. In a large skillet, heat the olive oil over medium heat. Add the diced onion, carrots, celery, and garlic. Cook until the vegetables are softened, about 5-7 minutes.

3. Add the cooked lentils, frozen peas, corn kernels, tomato paste, vegetable broth, and Worcestershire sauce (if using) to the skillet. Season with salt and pepper to taste. Cook for an additional 5 minutes, allowing the flavors to meld.

4. Transfer the lentil and vegetable mixture to the prepared baking dish. Spread the mashed potatoes evenly over the top.

5. Bake in the preheated oven for 25-30 minutes, or until the shepherd's pie is heated through and the mashed potatoes are lightly golden on top.

6. Serve the Lentil and Vegetable Shepherd's Pie hot, garnished with chopped parsley if desired.

Time Frame: Prep Time: 15 minutes, Cook Time: 35-40 minutes, Total Time: 50-55 minutes

Nutritional Information (per serving):

- Calories: 320 kcal
- Total Fat: 5 g
- Saturated Fat: 1 g
- Cholesterol: 0 mg
- Sodium: 280 mg
- Total Carbohydrates: 58 g
- Dietary Fiber: 13 g
- Sugars: 10 g
- Protein: 13 g

3. Creamy Butternut Squash Risotto:

Ingredients:
- 1 small butternut squash, peeled, seeded, and diced
- 2 tablespoons olive oil
- 1 onion, diced
- 2 cloves garlic, minced
- 1 ½ cups Arborio rice
- ½ cup dry white wine (optional)
- 4 cups vegetable broth, heated
- ½ cup grated Parmesan cheese (optional)
- Salt and pepper, to taste
- Fresh parsley, chopped (for garnish)

Instructions:
1. Preheat the oven to 400°F (200°C). Place the diced butternut squash on a baking sheet, drizzle with olive oil, and season with salt and pepper. Roast in the preheated oven for 20-25 minutes, or until tender.

2. In a large skillet, heat the remaining olive oil over medium heat. Add the diced onion and garlic, and sauté until softened, about 5 minutes.

3. Add the Arborio rice to the skillet and toast for 1-2 minutes, stirring constantly.

4. If using, pour in the white wine and cook until it has evaporated.

5. Gradually add the heated vegetable broth to the skillet, about 1 cup at a time, stirring frequently and allowing the liquid to absorb before adding more.

6. Once the risotto is creamy and the rice is cooked through (about 20-25 minutes), stir in the roasted butternut squash and grated Parmesan cheese (if using).

7. Season with additional salt and pepper to taste, if needed.

8. Serve the Creamy Butternut Squash Risotto hot, garnished with chopped fresh parsley.

Time Frame: Prep Time: 10 minutes, Cook Time: 45-50 minutes, Total Time: 55-60 minutes

Nutritional Information (per serving, without Parmesan cheese):
- Calories: 280 kcal
- Total Fat: 7 g
- Saturated Fat: 1 g
- Cholesterol: 0 mg
- Sodium: 480 mg
- Total Carbohydrates: 50 g
- Dietary Fiber: 4 g
- Sugars: 4 g
- Protein: 5 g

4. Spinach and Feta Stuffed Portobello Mushrooms:

Ingredients:
- 4 large Portobello mushrooms
- 2 tablespoons olive oil
- 2 cloves garlic, minced
- 2 cups fresh spinach, chopped

- ½ cup crumbled feta cheese
- Salt and pepper, to taste
- Fresh parsley, chopped (for garnish)

Instructions:
1. Preheat the oven to 375°F (190°C). Remove the stems from the Portobello mushrooms and gently scrape out the gills using a spoon. Place the mushrooms on a baking sheet lined with parchment paper.
2. In a skillet, heat the olive oil over medium heat. Add the minced garlic and cook until fragrant, about 1 minute.
3. Add the chopped spinach to the skillet and cook until wilted, about 2-3 minutes. Season with salt and pepper to taste.
4. Remove the skillet from the heat and stir in the crumbled feta cheese.
5. Divide the spinach and feta mixture evenly among the Portobello mushrooms, filling the hollowed-out centers.
6. Bake in the preheated oven for 15-20 minutes, or until the mushrooms are tender and the filling is heated through.
7. Serve the Spinach and Feta Stuffed Portobello Mushrooms hot, garnished with chopped fresh parsley.

Time Frame: Prep Time: 10 minutes, Cook Time: 15-20 minutes, Total Time: 25-30 minutes

Nutritional Information (per serving):
- Calories: 120 kcal
- Total Fat: 8 g
- Saturated Fat: 3 g
- Cholesterol: 15 mg
- Sodium: 260 mg
- Total Carbohydrates: 7 g
- Dietary Fiber: 2 g
- Sugars: 3 g

- Protein: 6 g

5. Veggie-Packed Minestrone Soup:

Ingredients:
- 2 tablespoons olive oil
- 1 onion, diced
- 2 carrots, diced
- 2 celery stalks, diced
- 2 cloves garlic, minced
- 1 can (15 oz) diced tomatoes
- 6 cups vegetable broth
- 1 can (15 oz) kidney beans, drained and rinsed
- 1 cup small pasta (e.g., ditalini, small shells)
- 2 cups chopped fresh spinach or kale
- 1 teaspoon dried basil
- 1 teaspoon dried oregano
- Salt and pepper, to taste
- Grated Parmesan cheese (for serving, optional)

Instructions:
1. In a large pot or Dutch oven, heat the olive oil over medium heat. Add the diced onion, carrots, celery, and garlic. Cook until the vegetables are softened, about 5-7 minutes.
2. Add the diced tomatoes (with their juices) to the pot, along with the vegetable broth. Bring the mixture to a boil.
3. Once boiling, reduce the heat to low and add the kidney beans, pasta, chopped spinach or kale, dried basil, and dried oregano. Simmer for 10-12 minutes, or until the pasta is cooked and the vegetables are tender.
4. Season the soup with salt and pepper to taste.
5. Serve the Veggie-Packed Minestrone Soup hot, garnished with grated Parmesan cheese if desired.

Time Frame: Prep Time: 10 minutes, Cook Time: 20-25 minutes, Total Time: 30-35 minutes

Nutritional Information (per serving, without Parmesan cheese):
- Calories: 220 kcal
- Total Fat: 6 g
- Saturated Fat: 1 g
- Cholesterol: 0 mg
- Sodium: 600 mg
- Total Carbohydrates: 35 g
- Dietary Fiber: 7 g
- Sugars: 6 g
- Protein: 9 g

6. Eggplant Parmesan Casserole:

Ingredients:
- 2 large eggplants, sliced into ½-inch rounds
- 2 cups marinara sauce
- 2 cups shredded mozzarella cheese
- ½ cup grated Parmesan cheese
- ½ cup breadcrumbs (optional)
- 2 tablespoons olive oil
- Salt and pepper, to taste
- Fresh basil leaves (for garnish)

Instructions:
1. Preheat the oven to 375°F (190°C). Grease a baking dish with olive oil or cooking spray.
2. Arrange the sliced eggplants in a single layer on a baking sheet. Brush both sides of the eggplant slices with olive oil and season with salt and pepper.

3. Bake the eggplant slices in the preheated oven for 20-25 minutes, or until they are tender and lightly browned.

4. Spread a thin layer of marinara sauce on the bottom of the prepared baking dish. Place a layer of baked eggplant slices on top of the sauce.

5. Sprinkle a layer of shredded mozzarella cheese and grated Parmesan cheese over the eggplant slices.

6. Repeat the layers until all of the ingredients are used, finishing with a layer of cheese on top.

7. If desired, sprinkle breadcrumbs over the top of the casserole for added texture.

8. Bake the Eggplant Parmesan Casserole in the preheated oven for 25-30 minutes, or until the cheese is melted and bubbly.

9. Remove the casserole from the oven and let it cool for a few minutes before serving.

10. Garnish with fresh basil leaves before serving.

Time Frame: Prep Time: 15 minutes, Cook Time: 50-55 minutes, Total Time: 65-70 minutes

Nutritional Information (per serving):
- Calories: 280 kcal
- Total Fat: 15 g
- Saturated Fat: 7 g
- Cholesterol: 30 mg
- Sodium: 700 mg
- Total Carbohydrates: 21 g
- Dietary Fiber: 6 g
- Sugars: 9 g
- Protein: 16 g

7. Chickpea and Sweet Potato Curry:

Ingredients:
- 2 tablespoons olive oil
- 1 onion, diced
- 2 cloves garlic, minced
- 1 tablespoon grated fresh ginger
- 2 sweet potatoes, peeled and diced
- 1 can (15 oz) chickpeas, drained and rinsed
- 1 can (14 oz) coconut milk
- 1 can (14 oz) diced tomatoes
- 2 tablespoons curry powder
- 1 teaspoon ground cumin
- Salt and pepper, to taste
- Fresh cilantro leaves (for garnish)
- Cooked rice, for serving

Instructions:
1. In a large skillet or pot, heat the olive oil over medium heat. Add the diced onion and cook until softened, about 5 minutes.
2. Add the minced garlic and grated ginger to the skillet and cook for an additional 1-2 minutes, until fragrant.
3. Stir in the diced sweet potatoes, chickpeas, coconut milk, diced tomatoes, curry powder, and ground cumin. Season with salt and pepper to taste.
4. Bring the mixture to a simmer, then reduce the heat to low. Cover and cook for 20-25 minutes, or until the sweet potatoes are tender.
5. Serve the Chickpea and Sweet Potato Curry hot, garnished with fresh cilantro leaves. Serve over cooked rice.

Time Frame: Prep Time: 10 minutes, Cook Time: 30-35 minutes, Total Time: 40-45 minutes

Nutritional Information (per serving, without rice):
- Calories: 320 kcal

- Total Fat: 15 g
- Saturated Fat: 8 g
- Cholesterol: 0 mg
- Sodium: 560 mg
- Total Carbohydrates: 40 g
- Dietary Fiber: 9 g
- Sugars: 11 g
- Protein: 8 g

8. Caprese Pasta Salad with Balsamic Glaze:

Ingredients:
- 8 oz (about 2 cups) pasta (such as penne or fusilli)
- 1 cup cherry tomatoes, halved
- 1 cup fresh mozzarella balls (ciliegine), halved
- ½ cup fresh basil leaves, torn
- 2 tablespoons balsamic glaze
- 2 tablespoons extra virgin olive oil
- Salt and pepper, to taste

Instructions:
1. Cook the pasta according to the package instructions until al dente. Drain and rinse under cold water to cool.
2. In a large bowl, combine the cooked pasta, cherry tomatoes, fresh mozzarella balls, and torn basil leaves.
3. Drizzle the balsamic glaze and extra virgin olive oil over the pasta salad. Season with salt and pepper to taste.
4. Toss gently to combine all the ingredients.
5. Serve the Caprese Pasta Salad chilled or at room temperature.

Time Frame: Prep Time: 10 minutes, Cook Time: 10-12 minutes, Total Time: 20-25 minutes

Nutritional Information (per serving):
- Calories: 300 kcal
- Total Fat: 12 g
- Saturated Fat: 4 g
- Cholesterol: 20 mg
- Sodium: 240 mg
- Total Carbohydrates: 35 g
- Dietary Fiber: 2 g
- Sugars: 3 g
- Protein: 12 g

9. Cauliflower Crust Margherita Pizza:

Ingredients:
- 1 medium cauliflower head, grated (about 4 cups)
- 1 egg, beaten
- ½ cup grated Parmesan cheese
- 1 teaspoon dried oregano
- 1 teaspoon garlic powder
- Salt and pepper, to taste
- ½ cup marinara sauce
- 1 cup shredded mozzarella cheese
- Fresh basil leaves, torn (for garnish)

Instructions:
1. Preheat the oven to 400°F (200°C). Line a baking sheet with parchment paper.
2. Place the grated cauliflower in a microwave-safe bowl and microwave on high for 5-6 minutes, or until softened.
3. Allow the cauliflower to cool slightly, then transfer it to a clean kitchen towel. Squeeze out as much excess moisture as possible.

4. In a large mixing bowl, combine the squeezed cauliflower, beaten egg, grated Parmesan cheese, dried oregano, garlic powder, salt, and pepper. Mix until well combined.

5. Transfer the cauliflower mixture to the prepared baking sheet and press it into a round crust shape, about ¼-inch thick.

6. Bake the cauliflower crust in the preheated oven for 20-25 minutes, or until golden brown and firm.

7. Remove the crust from the oven and spread the marinara sauce evenly over the surface.

8. Sprinkle the shredded mozzarella cheese over the sauce.

9. Return the pizza to the oven and bake for an additional 5-7 minutes, or until the cheese is melted and bubbly.

10. Garnish the Cauliflower Crust Margherita Pizza with torn fresh basil leaves before serving.

Time Frame: Prep Time: 15 minutes, Cook Time: 30-32 minutes, Total Time: 45-47 minutes

Nutritional Information (per serving):
- Calories: 220 kcal
- Total Fat: 12 g
- Saturated Fat: 6 g
- Cholesterol: 65 mg
- Sodium: 450 mg
- Total Carbohydrates: 14 g
- Dietary Fiber: 5 g
- Sugars: 4 g
- Protein: 17 g

10. Zucchini Noodles with Pesto and Cherry Tomatoes:

Ingredients:

- 4 medium zucchini, spiralized into noodles
- 1 cup cherry tomatoes, halved
- ¼ cup store-bought or homemade pesto sauce
- 2 tablespoons grated Parmesan cheese (optional)
- Salt and pepper, to taste
- Fresh basil leaves, torn (for garnish)

Instructions:
1. Heat a large skillet over medium heat. Add the zucchini noodles and cherry tomatoes to the skillet. Cook for 3-4 minutes, stirring occasionally, until the noodles are tender and the tomatoes are slightly softened.
2. Remove the skillet from the heat and stir in the pesto sauce until the noodles and tomatoes are evenly coated.
3. Season with salt and pepper to taste.
4. Serve the Zucchini Noodles with Pesto and Cherry Tomatoes hot, garnished with grated Parmesan cheese (if using) and torn fresh basil leaves.

Time Frame: Prep Time: 10 minutes, Cook Time: 5-7 minutes, Total Time: 15-17 minutes

Nutritional Information (per serving, without Parmesan cheese):
- Calories: 120 kcal
- Total Fat: 9 g
- Saturated Fat: 1.5 g
- Cholesterol: 0 mg
- Sodium: 180 mg
- Total Carbohydrates: 8 g
- Dietary Fiber: 3 g
- Sugars: 5 g
- Protein: 3 g

One-Pot Wonders for Easy Cleanup

1. One-Pot Chicken and Rice Casserole:

Ingredients:
- 1 tablespoon olive oil
- 1 onion, diced
- 2 cloves garlic, minced
- 2 boneless, skinless chicken breasts, diced
- 1 cup long-grain white rice
- 2 cups low-sodium chicken broth
- 1 cup frozen mixed vegetables
- 1 teaspoon dried thyme
- Salt and pepper to taste
- 1/4 cup grated Parmesan cheese (optional)

Instructions:
1. In a large skillet or pot, heat olive oil over medium heat. Add diced onion and minced garlic, sauté until softened.
2. Add diced chicken breasts to the skillet, cook until browned on all sides.
3. Stir in long-grain white rice, chicken broth, frozen mixed vegetables, dried thyme, salt, and pepper.
4. Bring the mixture to a boil, then reduce heat to low. Cover and simmer for 20-25 minutes, or until the rice is cooked and the liquid is absorbed.
5. If desired, sprinkle grated Parmesan cheese over the top before serving.

Time frame: Approximately 35 minutes
Nutritional information (per serving):
- Calories: 320 kcal
- Protein: 25g
- Carbohydrates: 30g
- Fat: 10g

- Fiber: 3g

2. Hearty Beef and Vegetable Stew:

Ingredients:
- 1 tablespoon olive oil
- 1 onion, diced
- 2 cloves garlic, minced
- 1 lb beef stew meat, cubed
- 4 cups low-sodium beef broth
- 2 carrots, sliced
- 2 potatoes, diced
- 1 cup frozen peas
- 1 teaspoon dried rosemary
- Salt and pepper to taste

Instructions:
1. Heat olive oil in a large pot over medium heat. Add diced onion and minced garlic, cook until fragrant.
2. Add cubed beef stew meat to the pot, brown on all sides.
3. Pour in low-sodium beef broth and bring to a boil.
4. Stir in sliced carrots, diced potatoes, frozen peas, dried rosemary, salt, and pepper.
5. Reduce heat to low, cover, and simmer for 1.5 to 2 hours, or until beef is tender.

Time frame: Approximately 2 hours and 30 minutes
Nutritional information (per serving):
- Calories: 350 kcal
- Protein: 25g
- Carbohydrates: 25g
- Fat: 15g

- Fiber: 5g

3. Creamy Mushroom Risotto with Peas:

Ingredients:
- 2 tablespoons olive oil
- 1 onion, finely chopped
- 2 cloves garlic, minced
- 1 1/2 cups Arborio rice
- 1/2 cup dry white wine (optional)
- 4 cups low-sodium vegetable broth
- 8 ounces cremini mushrooms, sliced
- 1 cup frozen peas
- 1/4 cup grated Parmesan cheese
- Salt and pepper to taste
- Fresh parsley, chopped (for garnish)

Instructions:
1. In a large skillet or pot, heat olive oil over medium heat. Add chopped onion and minced garlic, cook until softened.
2. Stir in Arborio rice and cook for 1-2 minutes until lightly toasted.
3. If using, pour in dry white wine and cook until it's absorbed.
4. Gradually add vegetable broth, about 1/2 cup at a time, stirring frequently and allowing the liquid to be absorbed before adding more.
5. When the rice is almost tender, stir in sliced cremini mushrooms and frozen peas. Continue cooking until the mushrooms are tender and the rice is creamy.
6. Remove from heat, stir in grated Parmesan cheese, and season with salt and pepper.
7. Garnish with chopped fresh parsley before serving.

Time frame: Approximately 40 minutes

Nutritional information (per serving):
- Calories: 320 kcal
- Protein: 8g
- Carbohydrates: 50g
- Fat: 8g
- Fiber: 5g

4. One-Pot Lemon Garlic Shrimp Pasta:

Ingredients:
- 8 ounces whole wheat spaghetti
- 1 tablespoon olive oil
- 2 cloves garlic, minced
- 1 lb large shrimp, peeled and deveined
- 2 cups low-sodium chicken broth
- 1 lemon, zest and juice
- 1/4 cup chopped fresh parsley
- Salt and pepper to taste
- Grated Parmesan cheese (optional)

Instructions:
1. In a large pot, cook whole wheat spaghetti according to package instructions until al dente. Drain and set aside.
2. In the same pot, heat olive oil over medium heat. Add minced garlic and cook until fragrant.
3. Add peeled and deveined shrimp to the pot, cook until pink and opaque.
4. Pour in low-sodium chicken broth, lemon zest, and lemon juice. Bring to a simmer.
5. Return cooked spaghetti to the pot, toss with shrimp and broth mixture until well combined.
6. Stir in chopped fresh parsley and season with salt and pepper.
7. Serve hot, garnished with grated Parmesan cheese if desired.

Time frame: Approximately 25 minutes
Nutritional information (per serving):
- Calories: 350 kcal
- Protein: 30g
- Carbohydrates: 40g
- Fat: 8g
- Fiber: 5g

5. Mexican Quinoa Skillet:

Ingredients:
- 1 tablespoon olive oil
- 1 onion, diced
- 2 cloves garlic, minced
- 1 bell pepper, diced
- 1 cup corn kernels (fresh or frozen)
- 1 cup black beans, drained and rinsed
- 1 cup quinoa, rinsed
- 1 can (14.5 oz) diced tomatoes
- 1 cup low-sodium vegetable broth
- 1 teaspoon chili powder
- 1/2 teaspoon cumin
- Salt and pepper to taste
- Fresh cilantro, chopped (for garnish)
- Avocado slices (for garnish)

Instructions:
1. Heat olive oil in a large skillet over medium heat. Add diced onion, minced garlic, and diced bell pepper, sauté until softened.
2. Stir in corn kernels, black beans, and quinoa, cook for 1-2 minutes.

3. Add diced tomatoes (with their juices), low-sodium vegetable broth, chili powder, cumin, salt, and pepper. Stir to combine.

4. Bring the mixture to a boil, then reduce heat to low. Cover and simmer for 15-20 minutes, or until quinoa is cooked and liquid is absorbed.

5. Remove from heat and let it sit, covered, for 5 minutes.

6. Fluff the quinoa with a fork and garnish with chopped fresh cilantro and avocado slices before serving.

Time frame: Approximately 30 minutes
Nutritional information (per serving):
- Calories: 300 kcal
- Protein: 10g
- Carbohydrates: 50g
- Fat: 7g
- Fiber: 10g

6. Tuscan White Bean Soup with Kale:

Ingredients:
- 1 tablespoon olive oil
- 1 onion, diced
- 2 cloves garlic, minced
- 2 carrots, diced
- 2 stalks celery, diced
- 4 cups low-sodium vegetable broth
- 2 cans (15 oz each) white beans, drained and rinsed
- 2 cups chopped kale leaves
- 1 teaspoon dried thyme
- Salt and pepper to taste
- Fresh lemon juice (optional, for serving)

Instructions:

1. Heat olive oil in a large pot over medium heat. Add diced onion, minced garlic, diced carrots, and diced celery, sauté until softened.

2. Pour in low-sodium vegetable broth and bring to a simmer.

3. Add drained and rinsed white beans, chopped kale leaves, dried thyme, salt, and pepper. Stir to combine.

4. Simmer for 15-20 minutes, or until the vegetables are tender and flavors are well combined.

5. Taste and adjust seasoning if needed. Squeeze fresh lemon juice over the soup before serving, if desired.

Time frame: Approximately 30 minutes
Nutritional information (per serving):
- Calories: 250 kcal
- Protein: 12g
- Carbohydrates: 40g
- Fat: 4g
- Fiber: 10g

7. Spicy Sausage and Pepper Pasta:

Ingredients:
- 8 ounces whole wheat penne pasta
- 1 tablespoon olive oil
- 1 onion, thinly sliced
- 2 cloves garlic, minced
- 8 ounces spicy Italian sausage, casings removed
- 1 bell pepper, thinly sliced
- 1 can (14.5 oz) diced tomatoes
- 1 teaspoon dried oregano
- 1/2 teaspoon red pepper flakes (adjust to taste)
- Salt and pepper to taste
- Grated Parmesan cheese (optional, for serving)

- Fresh basil leaves, torn (for garnish)

Instructions:
1. Cook whole wheat penne pasta according to package instructions until al dente. Drain and set aside.
2. In a large skillet, heat olive oil over medium heat. Add thinly sliced onion and minced garlic, cook until softened.
3. Add spicy Italian sausage to the skillet, breaking it into smaller pieces with a spatula. Cook until browned and cooked through.
4. Stir in thinly sliced bell pepper, diced tomatoes (with their juices), dried oregano, red pepper flakes, salt, and pepper. Simmer for 5-7 minutes.
5. Add cooked penne pasta to the skillet, toss with the sausage and pepper mixture until well combined.
6. Serve hot, garnished with grated Parmesan cheese and torn fresh basil leaves.

Time frame: Approximately 30 minutes
Nutritional information (per serving):
- Calories: 400 kcal
- Protein: 20g
- Carbohydrates: 40g
- Fat: 18g
- Fiber: 6g

8. Coconut Curry Lentil Soup:

Ingredients:
- 1 tablespoon coconut oil
- 1 onion, diced
- 2 cloves garlic, minced
- 1 tablespoon grated ginger
- 1 tablespoon curry powder

- 1 cup dried green lentils, rinsed
- 4 cups low-sodium vegetable broth
- 1 can (14 oz) coconut milk
- 2 carrots, diced
- 1 sweet potato, diced
- 2 cups chopped spinach
- Salt and pepper to taste
- Fresh cilantro, chopped (for garnish)
- Lime wedges (for serving)

Instructions:

1. In a large pot, heat coconut oil over medium heat. Add diced onion, minced garlic, grated ginger, and curry powder, sauté until fragrant.

2. Add rinsed green lentils and low-sodium vegetable broth to the pot, bring to a boil.

3. Reduce heat to low, stir in coconut milk, diced carrots, and diced sweet potato. Simmer for 20-25 minutes, or until lentils and vegetables are tender.

4. Stir in chopped spinach and cook until wilted. Season with salt and pepper to taste.

5. Serve hot, garnished with chopped fresh cilantro and lime wedges on the side.

Time frame: Approximately 40 minutes
Nutritional information (per serving):
- Calories: 350 kcal
- Protein: 15g
- Carbohydrates: 45g
- Fat: 12g
- Fiber: 12g

9. One-Pot Cajun Jambalaya:

Ingredients:
- 1 tablespoon olive oil
- 1 onion, diced
- 1 bell pepper, diced
- 2 celery stalks, diced
- 2 cloves garlic, minced
- 8 ounces Andouille sausage, sliced
- 1 cup long-grain white rice
- 1 can (14.5 oz) diced tomatoes
- 1 cup low-sodium chicken broth
- 1 teaspoon Cajun seasoning
- 1/2 teaspoon dried thyme
- 1 bay leaf
- 1 lb large shrimp, peeled and deveined
- Salt and pepper to taste
- Fresh parsley, chopped (for garnish)

Instructions:

1. In a large skillet or pot, heat olive oil over medium heat. Add diced onion, diced bell pepper, diced celery, and minced garlic, sauté until softened.

2. Add sliced Andouille sausage to the skillet, cook until browned.

3. Stir in long-grain white rice, diced tomatoes (with their juices), low-sodium chicken broth, Cajun seasoning, dried thyme, and bay leaf. Bring to a boil.

4. Reduce heat to low, cover, and simmer for 15-20 minutes, or until rice is cooked and liquid is absorbed.

5. Add peeled and deveined large shrimp to the pot, cook until pink and opaque.

6. Season with salt and pepper to taste, and garnish with chopped fresh parsley before serving.

Time frame: Approximately 40 minutes

Nutritional information (per serving):

- Calories: 400 kcal
- Protein: 25g
- Carbohydrates: 40g
- Fat: 15g
- Fiber: 5g

10. Mediterranean Orzo with Roasted Vegetables:

Ingredients:

- 1 cup orzo pasta
- 1 tablespoon olive oil
- 1 red bell pepper, diced
- 1 yellow bell pepper, diced
- 1 zucchini, diced
- 1 yellow squash, diced
- 1 red onion, diced
- 2 cloves garlic, minced
- 1 teaspoon dried oregano
- Salt and pepper to taste
- 1/4 cup crumbled feta cheese
- Fresh parsley, chopped (for garnish)
- Lemon wedges (for serving)

Instructions:

1. Preheat the oven to 400°F (200°C). Line a baking sheet with parchment paper.

2. In a large bowl, toss diced red bell pepper, diced yellow bell pepper, diced zucchini, diced yellow squash, diced red onion, minced garlic, dried oregano, olive oil, salt, and pepper until well coated.

3. Spread the vegetable mixture evenly on the prepared baking sheet. Roast in the preheated oven for 20-25 minutes, or until vegetables are tender and slightly caramelized.

4. In the meantime, cook orzo pasta according to package instructions until al dente. Drain and set aside.

5. Transfer the roasted vegetables to a large bowl, add cooked orzo pasta, and toss to combine.

6. Serve hot, garnished with crumbled feta cheese, chopped fresh parsley, and lemon wedges on the side.

Time frame: Approximately 40 minutes
Nutritional information (per serving):
- Calories: 350 kcal
- Protein: 10g
- Carbohydrates: 50g
- Fat: 10g
- Fiber: 8g

CHAPTER 5

WHOLESOME SIDE DISHES

Vibrant Vegetable Sides

1. Garlic Roasted Brussels Sprouts:
- **Ingredients:**
  - 1 lb Brussels sprouts, trimmed and halved
  - 2 tablespoons olive oil
  - 3 cloves garlic, minced
  - Salt and pepper to taste

Instructions:
1. Preheat the oven to 400°F (200°C).
2. In a large bowl, toss Brussels sprouts with olive oil, minced garlic, salt, and pepper until evenly coated.
3. Spread Brussels sprouts in a single layer on a baking sheet.
4. Roast in the preheated oven for 25-30 minutes, or until golden brown and tender, stirring halfway through.

Cooking time: 25-30 minutes
- **Nutritional information (per serving):**
  - Calories: 120
  - Total fat: 7g
  - Carbohydrates: 12g
  - Fiber: 5g
  - Protein: 4g

2. Lemon-Glazed Green Beans:
- **Ingredients:**

- 1 lb green beans, trimmed
- 2 tablespoons olive oil
- 2 tablespoons fresh lemon juice
- 1 teaspoon lemon zest
- Salt and pepper to taste

Instructions:

1. In a large skillet, heat olive oil over medium heat. Add green beans and sauté for 5-7 minutes, until tender-crisp.

2. Stir in lemon juice, lemon zest, salt, and pepper. Cook for an additional 2-3 minutes, until green beans are evenly coated and glazed.

Cooking time: 10-12 minutes

Nutritional information (per serving):
- Calories: 80
- Total fat: 5g
- Carbohydrates: 8g
- Fiber: 4g
- Protein: 2g

3. Honey-Glazed Carrots with Thyme:

Ingredients:
- 1 lb carrots, peeled and sliced into sticks
- 2 tablespoons honey
- 1 tablespoon olive oil
- 1 teaspoon fresh thyme leaves
- Salt and pepper to taste

Instructions:

1. Preheat the oven to 400°F (200°C).

2. In a large bowl, toss carrots with honey, olive oil, thyme leaves, salt, and pepper until evenly coated.

3. Spread carrots in a single layer on a baking sheet.

4. Roast in the preheated oven for 20-25 minutes, or until caramelized and tender, stirring halfway through.

Cooking time: 20-25 minutes

Nutritional information (per serving):

- Calories: 100
- Total fat: 3g
- Carbohydrates: 18g
- Fiber: 4g
- Protein: 1g

4. Ginger-Soy Glazed Bok Choy:

Ingredients:

- 4 baby bok choy, halved lengthwise
- 2 tablespoons soy sauce
- 1 tablespoon rice vinegar
- 1 tablespoon honey
- 1 teaspoon grated ginger
- 1 clove garlic, minced
- 1 tablespoon sesame oil

Instructions:

1. In a small bowl, whisk together soy sauce, rice vinegar, honey, grated ginger, minced garlic, and sesame oil.

2. Heat a large skillet over medium heat. Place bok choy in the skillet, cut side down.

3. Pour the soy sauce mixture over the bok choy. Cover and cook for 5-7 minutes, until bok choy is tender and glazed.

Cooking time: 5-7 minutes

Nutritional information (per serving):

- Calories: 70
- Total fat: 4g
- Carbohydrates: 8g
- Fiber: 2g
- Protein: 2g

5. Mediterranean Roasted Vegetables:
Ingredients:
- 1 lb mixed vegetables (such as bell peppers, zucchini, eggplant, cherry tomatoes)
- 2 tablespoons olive oil
- 2 cloves garlic, minced
- 1 teaspoon dried oregano
- Salt and pepper to taste

Instructions:
1. Preheat the oven to 425°F (220°C).
2. In a large bowl, toss mixed vegetables with olive oil, minced garlic, dried oregano, salt, and pepper until evenly coated.
3. Spread vegetables in a single layer on a baking sheet.
4. Roast in the preheated oven for 25-30 minutes, or until vegetables are tender and lightly browned, stirring halfway through.

Cooking time: 25-30 minutes
Nutritional information (per serving):
- Calories: 90
- Total fat: 5g
- Carbohydrates: 10g
- Fiber: 4g
- Protein: 2g

6. Spicy Sautéed Spinach with Garlic:

Ingredients:
- 1 lb fresh spinach leaves
- 2 tablespoons olive oil
- 3 cloves garlic, minced
- 1/2 teaspoon red pepper flakes
- Salt and pepper to taste

Instructions:

1. Heat olive oil in a large skillet over medium heat. Add minced garlic and red pepper flakes. Cook for 1 minute, until garlic is fragrant.

2. Add spinach to the skillet in batches, stirring until wilted.

3. Season with salt and pepper to taste. Continue to cook for an additional 2-3 minutes, until spinach is tender.

Cooking time: 5-7 minutes

Nutritional information (per serving):
- Calories: 60
- Total fat: 5g
- Carbohydrates: 3g
- Fiber: 2g
- Protein: 2g

7. Maple-Roasted Sweet Potatoes and Butternut Squash:

Ingredients:
- 1 lb sweet potatoes, peeled and cubed
- 1 lb butternut squash, peeled and cubed
- 2 tablespoons maple syrup
- 2 tablespoons olive oil
- 1 teaspoon cinnamon
- Salt to taste

Instructions:

1. Preheat the oven to 400°F (200°C).
2. In a large bowl, toss sweet potatoes and butternut squash with maple syrup, olive oil, cinnamon, and salt until evenly coated.
3. Spread vegetables in a single layer on a baking sheet.
4. Roast in the preheated oven for 30-35 minutes, or until vegetables are caramelized and tender, stirring halfway through.

Cooking time: 30-35 minutes
Nutritional information (per serving):
   - Calories: 120
   - Total fat: 5g
   - Carbohydrates: 20g
   - Fiber: 4g
   - Protein: 2g

8. Grilled Asparagus with Parmesan:
   Ingredients:
   - 1 lb asparagus spears, trimmed
   - 2 tablespoons olive oil
   - 2 tablespoons grated Parmesan cheese
   - Salt and pepper to taste

Instructions:
1. Preheat grill to medium-high heat.
2. In a large bowl, toss asparagus spears with olive oil, grated Parmesan cheese, salt, and pepper until evenly coated.
3. Grill asparagus for 5-7 minutes, turning occasionally, until tender and lightly charred.

Cooking time: 5-7 minutes
Nutritional information (per serving):
   - Calories: 70

- Total fat: 5g
- Carbohydrates: 4g
- Fiber: 2g
- Protein: 3g

9. Turmeric-Roasted Cauliflower:
Ingredients:
- 1 head cauliflower, cut into florets
- 2 tablespoons olive oil
- 1 teaspoon ground turmeric
- 1/2 teaspoon ground cumin
- Salt and pepper to taste

Instructions:
1. Preheat the oven to 425°F (220°C).
2. In a large bowl, toss cauliflower florets with olive oil, ground turmeric, ground cumin, salt, and pepper until evenly coated.
3. Spread cauliflower in a single layer on a baking sheet.
4. Roast in the preheated oven for 20-25 minutes, or until cauliflower is golden brown and tender, stirring halfway through.

Cooking time: 20-25 minutes
Nutritional information (per serving):
- Calories: 60
- Total fat: 5g
- Carbohydrates: 5g
- Fiber: 3g
- Protein: 2g

10. Sesame-Ginger Broccoli Stir-Fry:
Ingredients:
- 1 lb broccoli florets

- 2 tablespoons sesame oil
- 2 tablespoons soy sauce
- 1 tablespoon rice vinegar
- 1 tablespoon honey
- 1 teaspoon grated ginger
- 2 cloves garlic, minced
- 2 tablespoons sesame seeds

Instructions:

1. Heat sesame oil in a large skillet or wok over medium-high heat.

2. Add minced garlic and grated ginger to the skillet. Stir-fry for 1 minute until fragrant.

3. Add broccoli florets to the skillet and stir-fry for 3-4 minutes, until tender-crisp.

4. In a small bowl, whisk together soy sauce, rice vinegar, and honey. Pour the mixture over the broccoli in the skillet and toss to coat evenly.

5. Sprinkle sesame seeds over the stir-fry and cook for an additional 1-2 minutes.

Cooking time: 7-9 minutes

Nutritional information (per serving):

- Calories: 90
- Total fat: 5g
- Carbohydrates: 10g
- Fiber: 4g
- Protein: 3g

Nutritious Grain and Legume Sides

1. Quinoa Pilaf with Herbs and Lemon:

Ingredients:

- 1 cup quinoa, rinsed
- 2 cups vegetable broth
- 1 tablespoon olive oil
- 2 cloves garlic, minced
- 1/4 cup chopped fresh parsley
- 2 tablespoons chopped fresh mint
- Zest and juice of 1 lemon
- Salt and pepper to taste

Instructions:

1. In a saucepan, bring the vegetable broth to a boil. Stir in the quinoa, reduce heat to low, cover, and simmer for 15-20 minutes, or until the quinoa is cooked and liquid is absorbed.

2. In a separate skillet, heat olive oil over medium heat. Add minced garlic and sauté until fragrant, about 1 minute.

3. Fluff cooked quinoa with a fork and transfer to a large mixing bowl.

4. Add sautéed garlic, chopped parsley, chopped mint, lemon zest, and lemon juice to the quinoa. Season with salt and pepper to taste. Toss until well combined.

5. Serve warm as a side dish or as a light main course.

Time frame: Approximately 25 minutes
Nutritional information (per serving):
- Calories: 210
- Protein: 5g
- Fat: 5g
- Carbohydrates: 35g
- Fiber: 4g

2. Lentil and Brown Rice Casserole:
Ingredients:
- 1 cup brown rice

- 1 cup green or brown lentils
- 4 cups vegetable broth
- 1 onion, diced
- 2 cloves garlic, minced
- 1 carrot, diced
- 1 celery stalk, diced
- 1 teaspoon dried thyme
- 1 teaspoon dried oregano
- Salt and pepper to taste

Instructions:
1. Preheat the oven to 375°F (190°C). Lightly grease a casserole dish.
2. In a large saucepan, combine brown rice, lentils, vegetable broth, diced onion, minced garlic, diced carrot, diced celery, dried thyme, and dried oregano. Bring to a boil.
3. Reduce heat, cover, and simmer for 35-40 minutes, or until rice and lentils are tender and liquid is absorbed.
4. Transfer the mixture to the prepared casserole dish. Season with salt and pepper to taste.
5. Bake in the preheated oven for 25-30 minutes, or until the top is golden brown.
6. Serve hot as a main dish or side dish.

Time frame: Approximately 1 hour 20 minutes
Nutritional information (per serving):
- Calories: 280
- Protein: 14g
- Fat: 1g
- Carbohydrates: 54g
- Fiber: 9g

3. Mediterranean Chickpea Salad:

Ingredients:
- 2 cups cooked chickpeas (or 1 can, drained and rinsed)
- 1 cucumber, diced
- 1 tomato, diced
- 1/4 cup chopped red onion
- 1/4 cup chopped fresh parsley
- 1/4 cup chopped fresh mint
- 1/4 cup crumbled feta cheese (optional)
- 2 tablespoons extra virgin olive oil
- 1 tablespoon lemon juice
- 1 teaspoon dried oregano
- Salt and pepper to taste

Instructions:
1. In a large mixing bowl, combine cooked chickpeas, diced cucumber, diced tomato, chopped red onion, chopped parsley, chopped mint, and crumbled feta cheese (if using).
2. In a small bowl, whisk together extra virgin olive oil, lemon juice, dried oregano, salt, and pepper.
3. Pour the dressing over the salad and toss until well combined.
4. Serve chilled or at room temperature as a refreshing side dish or light lunch.

Time frame: Approximately 15 minutes
Nutritional information (per serving):
- Calories: 230
- Protein: 9g
- Fat: 11g
- Carbohydrates: 26g
- Fiber: 7g

4. Wild Rice with Mushrooms and Herbs:

Ingredients:
- 1 cup wild rice
- 2 cups vegetable broth
- 1 tablespoon olive oil
- 8 ounces mushrooms, sliced
- 2 cloves garlic, minced
- 2 tablespoons chopped fresh thyme
- Salt and pepper to taste

Instructions:

1. In a saucepan, combine wild rice and vegetable broth. Bring to a boil, then reduce heat to low, cover, and simmer for 45-50 minutes, or until rice is tender and liquid is absorbed.

2. In a separate skillet, heat olive oil over medium heat. Add sliced mushrooms and sauté until browned and tender, about 5-7 minutes.

3. Add minced garlic and chopped fresh thyme to the skillet with the mushrooms. Cook for an additional 1-2 minutes, until garlic is fragrant.

4. Fluff cooked wild rice with a fork and transfer to a serving bowl. Add sautéed mushrooms, garlic, and thyme. Season with salt and pepper to taste. Toss until well combined.

5. Serve hot as a hearty side dish or as a base for grilled or roasted proteins.

Time frame: Approximately 1 hour
Nutritional information (per serving):
- Calories: 210
- Protein: 6g
- Fat: 5g
- Carbohydrates: 35g
- Fiber: 4g

5. Bulgur Wheat Tabbouleh:
Ingredients:

- 1 cup bulgur wheat
- 2 cups boiling water
- 1 cucumber, diced
- 2 tomatoes, diced
- 1/2 red onion, finely chopped
- 1/4 cup chopped fresh parsley
- 1/4 cup chopped fresh mint
- 1/4 cup lemon juice
- 2 tablespoons extra virgin olive oil
- Salt and pepper to taste

Instructions:

1. Place bulgur wheat in a heatproof bowl. Pour boiling water over the bulgur wheat, cover, and let sit for 20-25 minutes, or until bulgur is tender and water is absorbed. Fluff with a fork.

2. In a large mixing bowl, combine cooked bulgur wheat, diced cucumber, diced tomatoes, chopped red onion, chopped parsley, and chopped mint.

3. In a small bowl, whisk together lemon juice, extra virgin olive oil, salt, and pepper.

4. Pour the dressing over the bulgur wheat mixture and toss until well combined.

5. Serve chilled or at room temperature as a refreshing salad or side dish.

Time frame: Approximately 30 minutes

Nutritional information (per serving):

- Calories: 190
- Protein: 5g
- Fat: 7g
- Carbohydrates: 29g
- Fiber: 7g

6. Black Bean and Corn Salsa:

Ingredients:
- 1 can (15 ounces) black beans, drained and rinsed
- 1 cup frozen corn, thawed
- 1 red bell pepper, diced
- 1/2 red onion, finely chopped
- 1 jalapeño pepper, seeded and minced
- 1/4 cup chopped fresh cilantro
- 2 tablespoons lime juice
- 1 tablespoon extra virgin olive oil
- 1 teaspoon ground cumin
- Salt and pepper to taste

Instructions:
1. In a large mixing bowl, combine black beans, thawed corn, diced red bell pepper, finely chopped red onion, minced jalapeño pepper, and chopped cilantro.
2. In a small bowl, whisk together lime juice, extra virgin olive oil, ground cumin, salt, and pepper.
3. Pour the dressing over the black bean and corn mixture and toss until well combined.
4. Serve chilled or at room temperature as a flavorful salsa with tortilla chips, or as a topping for grilled proteins.

Time frame: Approximately 15 minutes
Nutritional information (per serving):
- Calories: 150
- Protein: 6g
- Fat: 3g
- Carbohydrates: 27g
- Fiber: 6g

7. Farro Salad with Roasted Vegetables:

Ingredients:
- 1 cup farro
- 2 cups vegetable broth
- 1 cup cherry tomatoes, halved
- 1 zucchini, diced
- 1 yellow squash, diced
- 1 red bell pepper, diced
- 1/4 cup chopped fresh basil
- 2 tablespoons balsamic vinegar
- 2 tablespoons extra virgin olive oil
- Salt and pepper to taste

Instructions:
1. Preheat the oven to 400°F (200°C). Line a baking sheet with parchment paper.
2. In a saucepan, combine farro and vegetable broth. Bring to a boil, then reduce heat to low, cover, and simmer for 25-30 minutes, or until farro is tender and liquid is absorbed.
3. While the farro is cooking, spread cherry tomatoes, diced zucchini, diced yellow squash, and diced red bell pepper on the prepared baking sheet. Drizzle with olive oil and season with salt and pepper to taste. Roast in the preheated oven for 20-25 minutes, or until vegetables are tender and lightly browned.
4. In a large mixing bowl, combine cooked farro, roasted vegetables, chopped fresh basil, balsamic vinegar, and extra virgin olive oil. Toss until well combined.
5. Serve chilled or at room temperature as a hearty salad or side dish.

Time frame: Approximately 1 hour
Nutritional information (per serving):
- Calories: 250
- Protein: 6g

- Fat: 6g
- Carbohydrates: 43g
- Fiber: 7g

8. Couscous with Roasted Garlic and Tomatoes:
Ingredients:
- 1 cup couscous
- 1 cup vegetable broth
- 1 head garlic
- 1 cup cherry tomatoes
- 2 tablespoons extra virgin olive oil
- 1 tablespoon balsamic vinegar
- Salt and pepper to taste
- Chopped fresh parsley for garnish

Instructions:
1. Preheat the oven to 400°F (200°C).
2. Cut the top off the head of garlic to expose the cloves. Drizzle with olive oil and wrap in aluminum foil. Place on a baking sheet.
3. Place cherry tomatoes on the same baking sheet. Drizzle with olive oil and season with salt and pepper to taste.
4. Roast garlic and tomatoes in the preheated oven for 25-30 minutes, or until garlic is tender and tomatoes are bursting.
5. In a saucepan, bring vegetable broth to a boil. Stir in couscous, cover, and remove from heat. Let sit for 5 minutes, then fluff with a fork.
6. Squeeze roasted garlic cloves out of their skins and mash into a paste. In a large mixing bowl, combine cooked couscous, roasted garlic paste, roasted cherry tomatoes, balsamic vinegar, and extra virgin olive oil. Season with salt and pepper to taste.
7. Garnish with chopped fresh parsley before serving.

Time frame: Approximately 45 minutes

Nutritional information (per serving):
- Calories: 220
- Protein: 5g
- Fat: 5g
- Carbohydrates: 39g
- Fiber: 4g

9. Barley and Vegetable Stir-Fry:
Ingredients:
- 1 cup barley
- 2 cups vegetable broth
- 1 tablespoon sesame oil
- 1 onion, thinly sliced
- 2 carrots, julienned
- 1 bell pepper, thinly sliced
- 1 cup snap peas
- 2 cloves garlic, minced
- 2 tablespoons soy sauce
- 1 tablespoon rice vinegar
- 1 teaspoon grated ginger
- 1 tablespoon sesame seeds
- Chopped green onions for garnish

Instructions:
1. In a saucepan, bring vegetable broth to a boil. Stir in barley, reduce heat to low, cover, and simmer for 30-35 minutes, or until barley is tender and liquid is absorbed.
2. In a large skillet or wok, heat sesame oil over medium-high heat. Add sliced onion, julienned carrots, thinly sliced bell pepper, and snap peas. Stir-fry for 5-7 minutes, or until vegetables are tender-crisp.
3. Add minced garlic to the skillet and stir-fry for an additional 1-2 minutes, until fragrant.

4. In a small bowl, whisk together soy sauce, rice vinegar, and grated ginger.

5. Add cooked barley to the skillet with the vegetables. Pour the soy sauce mixture over the barley and vegetables. Toss until well combined and heated through.

6. Serve hot, garnished with sesame seeds and chopped green onions.

Time frame: Approximately 45 minutes
Nutritional information (per serving):
- Calories: 280
- Protein: 7g
- Fat: 5g
- Carbohydrates: 54g
- Fiber: 10g

10. Red Lentil Curry with Coconut Milk:

Ingredients:
- 1 cup red lentils
- 3 cups vegetable broth
- 1 tablespoon coconut oil
- 1 onion, diced
- 2 cloves garlic, minced
- 1 tablespoon grated ginger
- 1 tablespoon curry powder
- 1 teaspoon ground turmeric
- 1 can (14 ounces) coconut milk
- Salt and pepper to taste
- Chopped fresh cilantro for garnish

Instructions:

1. In a saucepan, combine red lentils and vegetable broth. Bring to a boil, then reduce heat to low, cover, and simmer for 20-25 minutes, or until lentils are tender and liquid is absorbed.

2. In a separate skillet, heat coconut oil over medium heat. Add diced onion and sauté until translucent, about 5-7 minutes.

3. Add minced garlic, grated ginger, curry powder, and ground turmeric to the skillet with the onions. Cook for an additional 1-2 minutes, until fragrant.

4. Add cooked red lentils to the skillet with the onion mixture. Stir in coconut milk and simmer for 5-10 minutes, until heated through and flavors are blended.

5. Season with salt and pepper to taste. Garnish with chopped fresh cilantro before serving.

6. Serve hot with steamed rice or naan bread.

Time frame: Approximately 40 minutes

Nutritional information (per serving):

- Calories: 320

- Protein: 15g

- Fat: 15g

- Carbohydrates: 35g

- Fiber: 15g

Potato Alternatives for Kidney Health

1. Mashed Cauliflower with Garlic and Herbs:

Ingredients:

- 1 head cauliflower, chopped into florets

- 2 cloves garlic, minced

- 2 tablespoons olive oil

- 2 tablespoons chopped fresh herbs (such as parsley, thyme, or rosemary)

- Salt and pepper to taste

Instructions:

1. In a large pot, bring water to a boil. Add the cauliflower florets and cook for 8-10 minutes, or until tender.
2. Drain the cauliflower and transfer it to a food processor.
3. Add minced garlic, olive oil, and chopped herbs to the food processor.
4. Blend until smooth and creamy, scraping down the sides as needed.
5. Season with salt and pepper to taste.
6. Serve hot as a delicious alternative to mashed potatoes.

Time frame: Approximately 20 minutes
Nutritional information:
- Serving size: 1/2 cup
- Calories: 90
- Total Fat: 6g
- Total Carbohydrates: 8g
- Dietary Fiber: 4g
- Protein: 3g

2. Baked Sweet Potato Wedges:

Ingredients:
- 2 large sweet potatoes, washed and cut into wedges
- 2 tablespoons olive oil
- 1 teaspoon smoked paprika
- 1 teaspoon garlic powder
- Salt and pepper to taste

Instructions:
1. Preheat the oven to 425°F (220°C). Line a baking sheet with parchment paper.
2. In a large bowl, toss sweet potato wedges with olive oil, smoked paprika, garlic powder, salt, and pepper until evenly coated.
3. Spread the wedges in a single layer on the prepared baking sheet.

4. Bake for 25-30 minutes, flipping halfway through, until the wedges are golden brown and crispy.
5. Serve hot as a nutritious side dish or snack.

Time frame: Approximately 35 minutes
Nutritional information:
- Serving size: 1/2 cup
- Calories: 110
- Total Fat: 5g
- Total Carbohydrates: 16g
- Dietary Fiber: 2g
- Protein: 1g

3. Rutabaga and Carrot Mash:

Ingredients:
- 1 large rutabaga, peeled and diced
- 2 large carrots, peeled and diced
- 2 tablespoons unsalted butter
- 1/4 cup low-fat milk or vegetable broth
- Salt and pepper to taste

Instructions:
1. Place rutabaga and carrots in a large pot and cover with water. Bring to a boil over high heat, then reduce heat to medium and simmer for 20-25 minutes, or until vegetables are tender.
2. Drain the vegetables and return them to the pot.
3. Add butter and milk or vegetable broth to the pot.
4. Mash the vegetables using a potato masher until smooth and creamy.
5. Season with salt and pepper to taste.
6. Serve hot as a delicious and nutritious alternative to mashed potatoes.

Time frame: Approximately 35 minutes
Nutritional information:
- Serving size: 1/2 cup
- Calories: 90
- Total Fat: 4g
- Total Carbohydrates: 13g
- Dietary Fiber: 4g
- Protein: 2g

4. Turnip Fries with Rosemary:

Ingredients:
- 2 large turnips, peeled and cut into fries
- 2 tablespoons olive oil
- 1 teaspoon dried rosemary
- Salt and pepper to taste

Instructions:
1. Preheat the oven to 425°F (220°C). Line a baking sheet with parchment paper.
2. In a large bowl, toss turnip fries with olive oil, dried rosemary, salt, and pepper until evenly coated.
3. Spread the fries in a single layer on the prepared baking sheet.
4. Bake for 20-25 minutes, flipping halfway through, until the fries are golden brown and crispy.
5. Serve hot as a nutritious and flavorful alternative to traditional French fries.

Time frame: Approximately 35 minutes
Nutritional information:
- Serving size: 1/2 cup
- Calories: 80

- Total Fat: 4g
- Total Carbohydrates: 10g
- Dietary Fiber: 3g
- Protein: 1g

5. Celeriac and Potato Gratin:

Ingredients:
- 1 large celeriac (celery root), peeled and thinly sliced
- 2 large potatoes, peeled and thinly sliced
- 1 cup low-sodium vegetable broth
- 1/2 cup grated Parmesan cheese
- 2 cloves garlic, minced
- 1 teaspoon dried thyme
- Salt and pepper to taste

Instructions:
1. Preheat the oven to 375°F (190°C). Grease a baking dish with olive oil or cooking spray.
2. Layer celeriac and potato slices in the prepared baking dish, alternating between the two.
3. In a small bowl, mix vegetable broth, minced garlic, dried thyme, salt, and pepper.
4. Pour the broth mixture over the layered vegetables.
5. Sprinkle grated Parmesan cheese on top.
6. Cover the baking dish with aluminum foil and bake for 45 minutes.
7. Remove the foil and bake for an additional 15-20 minutes, or until the top is golden brown and the vegetables are tender.
8. Let it cool for a few minutes before serving.

Time frame: Approximately 1 hour and 15 minutes
Nutritional information:

- Serving size: 1/2 cup
- Calories: 120
- Total Fat: 3g
- Total Carbohydrates: 20g
- Dietary Fiber: 3g
- Protein: 5g

6. Parsnip and Carrot Puree:

Ingredients:
- 2 large parsnips, peeled and chopped
- 2 large carrots, peeled and chopped
- 2 tablespoons unsalted butter
- 1/4 cup low-fat milk or vegetable broth
- Salt and pepper to taste

Instructions:
1. Place parsnips and carrots in a large pot and cover with water. Bring to a boil over high heat, then reduce heat to medium and simmer for 15-20 minutes, or until vegetables are tender.
2. Drain the vegetables and return them to the pot.
3. Add butter and milk or vegetable broth to the pot.
4. Use an immersion blender to puree the vegetables until smooth and creamy.
5. Season with salt and pepper to taste.
6. Serve hot as a nutritious and flavorful side dish.

Time frame: Approximately 30 minutes
Nutritional information:
- Serving size: 1/2 cup
- Calories: 110
- Total Fat: 5g

- Total Carbohydrates: 16g
- Dietary Fiber: 4g
- Protein: 2g

7. Jicama Home Fries:

Ingredients:
- 2 large jicama, peeled and cut into cubes
- 2 tablespoons olive oil
- 1 teaspoon paprika
- 1/2 teaspoon garlic powder
- Salt and pepper to taste

Instructions:
1. Preheat the oven to 425°F (220°C). Line a baking sheet with parchment paper.
2. In a large bowl, toss jicama cubes with olive oil, paprika, garlic powder, salt, and pepper until evenly coated.
3. Spread the jicama cubes in a single layer on the prepared baking sheet.
4. Bake for 30-35 minutes, flipping halfway through, until the cubes are golden brown and crispy.
5. Serve hot as a nutritious and flavorful alternative to traditional home fries.

Time frame: Approximately 45 minutes
Nutritional information:
- Serving size: 1/2 cup
- Calories: 90
- Total Fat: 5g
- Total Carbohydrates: 12g
- Dietary Fiber: 6g
- Protein: 1g

8. Butternut Squash and Apple Hash:

Ingredients:
- 1 small butternut squash, peeled and diced
- 2 apples, peeled and diced
- 1 onion, diced
- 2 tablespoons olive oil
- 1 teaspoon ground cinnamon
- Salt and pepper to taste

Instructions:
1. Heat olive oil in a large skillet over medium heat.
2. Add diced butternut squash, apples, and onion to the skillet.
3. Sprinkle ground cinnamon, salt, and pepper over the mixture.
4. Cook, stirring occasionally, for 15-20 minutes, or until the squash is tender and caramelized.
5. Serve hot as a delicious and nutritious side dish or breakfast hash.

Time frame: Approximately 25 minutes
Nutritional information:
- Serving size: 1/2 cup
- Calories: 100
- Total Fat: 5g
- Total Carbohydrates: 15g
- Dietary Fiber: 4g
- Protein: 1g

9. Zucchini and Squash Casserole:

Ingredients:
- 2 zucchinis, sliced
- 2 yellow squashes, sliced

- 1 onion, thinly sliced
- 1 cup shredded low-fat mozzarella cheese
- 1/4 cup grated Parmesan cheese
- 2 cloves garlic, minced
- 1 teaspoon dried Italian herbs
- Salt and pepper to taste
- Olive oil cooking spray

Instructions:

1. Preheat the oven to 375°F (190°C). Grease a baking dish with olive oil cooking spray.

2. In a large bowl, combine sliced zucchinis, yellow squashes, and onions.

3. Add minced garlic, dried Italian herbs, salt, and pepper to the bowl. Toss until evenly coated.

4. Transfer the vegetable mixture to the prepared baking dish.

5. Sprinkle shredded mozzarella cheese and grated Parmesan cheese over the top.

6. Cover the baking dish with aluminum foil and bake for 25 minutes.

7. Remove the foil and bake for an additional 15-20 minutes, or until the cheese is melted and bubbly.

8. Serve hot as a nutritious and flavorful side dish.

Time frame: Approximately 50 minutes
Nutritional information:
- Serving size: 1/2 cup
- Calories: 90
- Total Fat: 4g
- Total Carbohydrates: 10g
- Dietary Fiber: 3g
- Protein: 6g

10. Spaghetti Squash with Tomato-Basil Sauce:

Ingredients:
- 1 spaghetti squash
- 2 cups tomato sauce (low-sodium)
- 1/4 cup chopped fresh basil leaves
- 2 cloves garlic, minced
- 1 tablespoon olive oil
- Salt and pepper to taste
- Grated Parmesan cheese for serving (optional)

Instructions:
1. Preheat the oven to 400°F (200°C). Cut the spaghetti squash in half lengthwise and scoop out the seeds.
2. Place the squash halves cut side down on a baking sheet lined with parchment paper.
3. Bake for 40-45 minutes, or until the squash is tender and easily pierced with a fork.
4. While the squash is baking, heat olive oil in a saucepan over medium heat. Add minced garlic and sauté for 1-2 minutes, or until fragrant.
5. Add tomato sauce to the saucepan and bring to a simmer. Cook for 10-15 minutes, stirring occasionally.
6. Stir in chopped basil leaves, salt, and pepper to taste.
7. Once the squash is done baking, use a fork to scrape the flesh into spaghetti-like strands.
8. Serve the spaghetti squash topped with tomato-basil sauce and grated Parmesan cheese, if desired.

Time frame: Approximately 1 hour and 5 minutes
Nutritional information:
- Serving size: 1 cup
- Calories: 110
- Total Fat: 3g

- Total Carbohydrates: 20g
- Dietary Fiber: 4g
- Protein: 2g

CHAPTER 6

SNACKS AND APPETIZERS

Quick and Easy Snacks on the Go

1. Nutty Energy Bites:

Ingredients:
- 1 cup rolled oats
- 1/2 cup natural peanut butter
- 1/3 cup honey
- 1/4 cup chopped nuts (almonds, walnuts, or cashews)
- 1/4 cup ground flaxseed
- 1/4 cup mini chocolate chips (optional)
- 1 teaspoon vanilla extract

Instructions:
1. In a large mixing bowl, combine all ingredients until well mixed.
2. Roll the mixture into small balls, about 1 inch in diameter.
3. Place the energy bites on a baking sheet lined with parchment paper.
4. Chill in the refrigerator for at least 30 minutes before serving.
5. Store in an airtight container in the refrigerator for up to one week.

Time frame: 10 minutes preparation + 30 minutes chilling
Nutritional information (per serving - 1 energy bite):
- Calories: 100
- Protein: 3g
- Fat: 5g
- Carbohydrates: 12g
- Fiber: 2g

- Sugars: 6g

2. Greek Yogurt Parfait Cups:

Ingredients:
- 1 cup plain Greek yogurt
- 1/2 cup granola
- 1/2 cup mixed berries (strawberries, blueberries, raspberries)
- Honey or maple syrup, to taste (optional)

Instructions:
1. In individual serving cups or bowls, layer Greek yogurt, granola, and mixed berries.
2. Drizzle with honey or maple syrup if desired.
3. Serve immediately or refrigerate until ready to eat.

Time frame: 5 minutes preparation
Nutritional information (per serving):
- Calories: 250
- Protein: 15g
- Fat: 6g
- Carbohydrates: 35g
- Fiber: 4g
- Sugars: 15g

3. Veggie Sticks with Hummus:

Ingredients:
- Assorted vegetables (carrots, celery, bell peppers, cucumbers), cut into sticks
- 1 cup hummus

Instructions:

1. Arrange vegetable sticks on a platter.
2. Serve with hummus for dipping.

Time frame: 5 minutes preparation

Nutritional information (per serving):

- Calories: 100
- Protein: 5g
- Fat: 6g
- Carbohydrates: 10g
- Fiber: 4g
- Sugars: 2g

4. Trail Mix Popcorn Balls:

Ingredients:

- 6 cups popped popcorn
- 1/2 cup dried fruit (raisins, cranberries, apricots), chopped
- 1/2 cup mixed nuts (almonds, cashews, peanuts), chopped
- 1/4 cup honey or maple syrup
- 1/4 cup peanut butter

Instructions:

1. In a large mixing bowl, combine popcorn, dried fruit, and nuts.
2. In a small saucepan, heat honey and peanut butter over low heat until melted and well combined.
3. Pour the honey-peanut butter mixture over the popcorn mixture and stir until evenly coated.
4. Using damp hands, shape the mixture into balls and place on a baking sheet lined with parchment paper.
5. Let cool for 30 minutes before serving.

Time frame: 15 minutes preparation + 30 minutes cooling
Nutritional information (per serving - 1 popcorn ball):
- Calories: 150
- Protein: 4g
- Fat: 8g
- Carbohydrates: 18g
- Fiber: 2g
- Sugars: 10g

5. Cheese and Whole Grain Crackers:

Ingredients:
- Assorted whole grain crackers
- Assorted low-fat cheese slices or cubes (cheddar, Swiss, mozzarella)

Instructions:
1. Arrange crackers and cheese on a platter.
2. Serve immediately.

Time frame: 5 minutes preparation
Nutritional information (per serving):
- Calories: 120
- Protein: 6g
- Fat: 5g
- Carbohydrates: 15g
- Fiber: 3g
- Sugars: 1g

6. Apple Slices with Almond Butter:

Ingredients:
- 2 apples, sliced

- 1/4 cup almond butter

Instructions:
1. Arrange apple slices on a plate.
2. Serve with almond butter for dipping or spreading.

Time frame: 5 minutes preparation
Nutritional information (per serving):
- Calories: 200
- Protein: 4g
- Fat: 12g
- Carbohydrates: 20g
- Fiber: 6g
- Sugars: 14g

7. Protein-Packed Deviled Eggs:

Ingredients:
- 6 hard-boiled eggs, peeled and halved
- 3 tablespoons Greek yogurt
- 1 tablespoon Dijon mustard
- Salt and pepper, to taste
- Paprika, for garnish

Instructions:
1. Remove egg yolks and place them in a mixing bowl.
2. Mash the egg yolks with Greek yogurt, Dijon mustard, salt, and pepper until smooth.
3. Spoon the mixture back into the egg white halves.
4. Sprinkle with paprika for garnish.
5. Chill in the refrigerator for at least 30 minutes before serving.

Time frame: 15 minutes preparation + 30 minutes chilling
Nutritional information (per serving - 2 egg halves):
- Calories: 120
- Protein: 10g
- Fat: 8g
- Carbohydrates: 2g
- Fiber: 0g
- Sugars: 1g

8. Banana-Oatmeal Muffins:

Ingredients:
- 2 ripe bananas, mashed
- 2 cups rolled oats
- 1/4 cup honey or maple syrup
- 1/4 cup milk (dairy or plant-based)
- 1 teaspoon vanilla extract
- 1 teaspoon ground cinnamon
- 1/2 teaspoon baking powder
- 1/4 teaspoon salt
- 1/4 cup chopped nuts (optional)

Instructions:
1. Preheat the oven to 350°F (175°C). Grease a muffin tin or line with paper liners.
2. In a large mixing bowl, combine mashed bananas, oats, honey or maple syrup, milk, vanilla extract, cinnamon, baking powder, salt, and chopped nuts (if using).
3. Divide the mixture evenly among the muffin cups.
4. Bake for 20-25 minutes, or until the muffins are golden brown and a toothpick inserted into the center comes out clean.
5. Let cool for 5 minutes before removing from the muffin tin.

Time frame: 10 minutes preparation + 25 minutes baking + 5 minutes cooling
Nutritional information (per muffin):
- Calories: 150
- Protein: 4g
- Fat: 3g
- Carbohydrates: 28g
- Fiber: 3g
- Sugars: 10g

9. Cottage Cheese and Fruit Cups:

Ingredients:
- 1 cup low-fat cottage cheese
- 1 cup mixed fruit (berries, grapes, melon), chopped

Instructions:
1. In individual serving cups or bowls, layer cottage cheese and mixed fruit.
2. Serve immediately or refrigerate until ready to eat.

Time frame: 5 minutes preparation
Nutritional information (per serving):
- Calories: 150
- Protein: 15g
- Fat: 2g
- Carbohydrates: 20g
- Fiber: 3g
- Sugars: 15g

10. Turkey and Cheese Roll-Ups:

Ingredients:
- 4 slices low-sodium turkey breast
- 4 slices low-fat cheese (cheddar, Swiss, mozzarella)
- 1/2 cup spinach leaves
- Mustard or mayonnaise, for spreading (optional)

Instructions:
1. Lay a slice of turkey breast on a flat surface.
2. Place a slice of cheese on top of the turkey.
3. Add spinach leaves on top of the cheese.
4. Roll up tightly and secure with toothpicks if necessary.
5. Repeat with the remaining ingredients.
6. Serve immediately or refrigerate until ready to eat.

Time frame: 5 minutes preparation
Nutritional information (per serving - 1 roll-up):
- Calories: 120
- Protein: 15g
- Fat: 5g
- Carbohydrates: 2g
- Fiber: 1g
- Sugars: 1g

Appetizers for Entertaining Seniors

1. Caprese Skewers with Balsamic Glaze:

Ingredients:
- 12 cherry tomatoes
- 12 fresh mozzarella balls
- 12 fresh basil leaves
- Balsamic glaze, for drizzling

- Salt and pepper to taste

Instructions:
1. Thread one cherry tomato, one mozzarella ball, and one basil leaf onto each skewer.
2. Arrange the skewers on a serving platter.
3. Drizzle with balsamic glaze and sprinkle with salt and pepper.
4. Serve immediately.

Time frame: Prep Time: 10 minutes
Total Time: 10 minutes

Nutritional information (per serving):
- Calories: 70kcal
- Fat: 5g
- Carbohydrates: 2g
- Protein: 4g

2. Mini Quiches with Spinach and Feta:

Ingredients:
- 6 large eggs
- 1/2 cup milk
- 1 cup chopped spinach
- 1/2 cup crumbled feta cheese
- Salt and pepper to taste
- Cooking spray

Instructions:
1. Preheat the oven to 350°F (175°C). Grease a mini muffin tin with cooking spray.

2. In a mixing bowl, whisk together the eggs and milk. Season with salt and pepper.

3. Stir in the chopped spinach and crumbled feta cheese.

4. Pour the egg mixture into the prepared muffin tin, filling each cup about 3/4 full.

5. Bake in the preheated oven for 12-15 minutes, or until the quiches are set and golden brown.

6. Allow the quiches to cool for a few minutes before serving.

Time frame: Prep Time: 10 minutes
Cook Time: 12-15 minutes
Total Time: 25 minutes

Nutritional information (per serving - 2 mini quiches):
- Calories: 120kcal
- Fat: 8g
- Carbohydrates: 2g
- Protein: 10g

3. Smoked Salmon Canapés on Cucumber Rounds:

Ingredients:
- 1 English cucumber, sliced into rounds
- 4 oz smoked salmon
- 1/4 cup cream cheese
- 2 tablespoons chopped fresh dill
- 1 tablespoon capers
- Lemon zest, for garnish

Instructions:
1. Arrange the cucumber rounds on a serving platter.
2. Spread a thin layer of cream cheese on each cucumber round.

3. Top each cucumber round with a piece of smoked salmon.
4. Sprinkle chopped fresh dill and capers over the smoked salmon.
5. Garnish with lemon zest.
6. Serve immediately.

Time frame: Prep Time: 10 minutes
            Total Time: 10 minutes

Nutritional information (per serving - 3 canapés):
- Calories: 90kcal
- Fat: 6g
- Carbohydrates: 2g
- Protein: 8g

4. Stuffed Mushrooms with Creamy Herb Filling:

Ingredients:
- 12 large button mushrooms
- 1/4 cup cream cheese, softened
- 2 tablespoons grated Parmesan cheese
- 1 tablespoon chopped fresh parsley
- 1 garlic clove, minced
- Salt and pepper to taste
- Olive oil, for brushing

Instructions:
1. Preheat the oven to 375°F (190°C). Line a baking sheet with parchment paper.
2. Remove the stems from the mushrooms and finely chop them.
3. In a mixing bowl, combine the chopped mushroom stems, cream cheese, Parmesan cheese, parsley, garlic, salt, and pepper.

4. Spoon the cream cheese mixture into the mushroom caps, dividing it evenly among them.

5. Place the stuffed mushrooms on the prepared baking sheet.

6. Lightly brush the tops of the mushrooms with olive oil.

7. Bake in the preheated oven for 15-20 minutes, or until the mushrooms are tender and the filling is golden brown.

8. Serve warm.

Time frame: Prep Time: 15 minutes
Cook Time: 15-20 minutes
Total Time: 30-35 minutes

Nutritional information (per serving - 3 stuffed mushrooms):
- Calories: 70kcal
- Fat: 5g
- Carbohydrates: 3g
- Protein: 3g

5. Shrimp Cocktail with Zesty Cocktail Sauce:

Ingredients:
- 12 large shrimp, cooked and peeled
- 1/2 cup ketchup
- 1 tablespoon prepared horseradish
- 1 tablespoon lemon juice
- 1 teaspoon Worcestershire sauce
- Hot sauce to taste (optional)
- Lemon wedges, for garnish
- Fresh parsley, for garnish

Instructions:

1. In a small bowl, mix together the ketchup, horseradish, lemon juice, Worcestershire sauce, and hot sauce (if using) to make the cocktail sauce.
2. Arrange the cooked shrimp on a serving platter.
3. Serve the shrimp with the zesty cocktail sauce on the side.
4. Garnish with lemon wedges and fresh parsley.
5. Serve chilled.

Time frame: Prep Time: 5 minutes
Total Time: 5 minutes

Nutritional information (per serving - 3 shrimp with sauce):
- Calories: 80kcal
- Fat: 1g
- Carbohydrates: 10g
- Protein: 8g

6. Chicken Satay Skewers with Peanut Dipping Sauce:

Ingredients:
- 1 lb boneless, skinless chicken breasts, cut into strips
- 1/4 cup soy sauce
- 2 tablespoons honey
- 1 tablespoon sesame oil
- 1 tablespoon lime juice
- 2 garlic cloves, minced
- 1 teaspoon ground coriander
- 1/2 teaspoon ground cumin
- Wooden skewers, soaked in water
- Chopped peanuts and chopped cilantro, for garnish (optional)

For Peanut Dipping Sauce:
- 1/4 cup creamy peanut butter

- 2 tablespoons soy sauce
- 1 tablespoon honey
- 1 tablespoon lime juice
- 1 teaspoon Sriracha sauce (optional)
- Water, as needed to thin the sauce

Instructions:

1. In a bowl, whisk together soy sauce, honey, sesame oil, lime juice, minced garlic, ground coriander, and ground cumin.

2. Add chicken strips to the marinade, cover, and refrigerate for at least 30 minutes, or up to 4 hours.

3. Preheat grill or grill pan over medium-high heat. Thread marinated chicken strips onto soaked wooden skewers.

4. Grill skewers for 4-5 minutes on each side, or until chicken is cooked through and nicely charred.

5. Meanwhile, prepare the peanut dipping sauce by whisking together peanut butter, soy sauce, honey, lime juice, and Sriracha sauce (if using). Add water as needed to achieve desired consistency.

6. Transfer grilled chicken satay skewers to a serving platter and garnish with chopped peanuts and cilantro, if desired.

7. Serve hot with peanut dipping sauce on the side.

Time frame: Prep Time: 10 minutes (plus marinating time)
        Cook Time: 10 minutes
        Total Time: 20 minutes (plus marinating time)

Nutritional information (per serving - 2 skewers with dipping sauce):
- Calories: 280kcal
- Fat: 14g
- Carbohydrates: 14g
- Protein: 26g

7. Bruschetta with Tomato and Basil:

Ingredients:
- 1 French baguette, sliced into 1/2-inch thick rounds
- 2 cups diced tomatoes
- 1/4 cup chopped fresh basil
- 2 garlic cloves, minced
- 2 tablespoons extra virgin olive oil
- 1 tablespoon balsamic vinegar
- Salt and pepper to taste

Instructions:
1. Preheat oven to 400°F (200°C). Place baguette slices on a baking sheet and lightly brush with olive oil. Toast in the oven for 5-7 minutes, or until golden brown and crispy.
2. In a mixing bowl, combine diced tomatoes, chopped basil, minced garlic, olive oil, and balsamic vinegar. Season with salt and pepper to taste.
3. Top each toasted baguette slice with the tomato-basil mixture.
4. Serve immediately, garnished with additional basil leaves if desired.

Time frame: Prep Time: 10 minutes
        Cook Time: 5-7 minutes
        Total Time: 15-17 minutes

Nutritional information (per serving - 2 bruschetta slices):
- Calories: 120kcal
- Fat: 5g
- Carbohydrates: 16g
- Protein: 3g

8. Baked Brie with Cranberry Chutney:

Ingredients:
- 1 round of Brie cheese
- 1/4 cup cranberry chutney (store-bought or homemade)
- 1/4 cup chopped pecans
- 1 tablespoon honey
- Crackers or bread slices, for serving

Instructions:
1. Preheat the oven to 350°F (175°C).
2. Place the Brie cheese on a baking sheet lined with parchment paper.
3. Spread the cranberry chutney over the top of the Brie.
4. Sprinkle chopped pecans on top of the cranberry chutney.
5. Drizzle honey over the pecans.
6. Bake in the preheated oven for 10-12 minutes, or until the Brie is soft and gooey.
7. Remove from the oven and let it cool for a few minutes before serving.
8. Serve with crackers or bread slices.

Time frame: Prep Time: 5 minutes
       Cook Time: 10-12 minutes
       Total Time: 15-17 minutes

Nutritional information (per serving - 2 tablespoons of baked Brie with cranberry chutney):
- Calories: 120kcal
- Fat: 9g
- Carbohydrates: 6g
- Protein: 5g

9. Prosciutto-Wrapped Asparagus Spears:

Ingredients:

- 12 asparagus spears, tough ends trimmed
- 6 slices prosciutto, halved lengthwise
- 1 tablespoon olive oil
- Salt and pepper to taste

Instructions:
1. Preheat the oven to 400°F (200°C).
2. Drizzle olive oil over the asparagus spears and toss to coat.
3. Season with salt and pepper.
4. Wrap each asparagus spear with a halved slice of prosciutto.
5. Place the prosciutto-wrapped asparagus spears on a baking sheet lined with parchment paper.
6. Bake in the preheated oven for 10-12 minutes, or until the asparagus is tender and the prosciutto is crispy.
7. Serve warm or at room temperature.

Time frame: Prep Time: 10 minutes
Cook Time: 10-12 minutes
Total Time: 20-22 minutes

Nutritional information (per serving - 3 prosciutto-wrapped asparagus spears):
- Calories: 90kcal
- Fat: 6g
- Carbohydrates: 2g
- Protein: 7g

10. Mini Meatballs in Marinara Sauce:

Ingredients:
For the meatballs:
- 1 lb ground beef or turkey

- 1/2 cup breadcrumbs
- 1/4 cup grated Parmesan cheese
- 1 egg
- 2 cloves garlic, minced
- 1 teaspoon dried oregano
- 1 teaspoon dried basil
- Salt and pepper to taste

For the marinara sauce:
- 1 tablespoon olive oil
- 1 small onion, diced
- 2 cloves garlic, minced
- 1 (14 oz) can crushed tomatoes
- 1 teaspoon dried oregano
- 1 teaspoon dried basil
- Salt and pepper to taste

Instructions:
1. Preheat the oven to 375°F (190°C). Line a baking sheet with parchment paper.
2. In a large bowl, combine ground meat, breadcrumbs, Parmesan cheese, egg, minced garlic, dried oregano, dried basil, salt, and pepper. Mix until well combined.
3. Roll the meat mixture into mini meatballs, about 1 inch in diameter, and place them on the prepared baking sheet.
4. Bake in the preheated oven for 15-20 minutes, or until the meatballs are cooked through and lightly browned.
5. While the meatballs are baking, prepare the marinara sauce. Heat olive oil in a saucepan over medium heat. Add diced onion and cook until softened, about 5 minutes. Add minced garlic and cook for an additional minute.

6. Stir in crushed tomatoes, dried oregano, dried basil, salt, and pepper. Simmer for 10-15 minutes, stirring occasionally, until the sauce has thickened slightly.

7. Once the meatballs are cooked, add them to the marinara sauce and toss to coat.

8. Serve the mini meatballs in marinara sauce with toothpicks for easy serving.

Time frame: Prep Time: 15 minutes
Cook Time: 30-35 minutes
Total Time: 45-50 minutes

Nutritional information (per serving - 4 mini meatballs with marinara sauce):
- Calories: 250kcal
- Fat: 12g
- Carbohydrates: 12g
- Protein: 20g

Dips and Spreads for Flavorful Nibbles

1. Creamy Avocado Dip with Lime:

Ingredients:
- 2 ripe avocados
- 1 lime, juiced
- 1/4 cup chopped cilantro
- 1/2 teaspoon garlic powder
- Salt and pepper to taste

Instructions:
1. Cut the avocados in half, remove the pit, and scoop the flesh into a bowl.

2. Mash the avocados with a fork until smooth.
3. Stir in the lime juice, chopped cilantro, garlic powder, salt, and pepper until well combined.
4. Serve immediately with your choice of chips or veggies.

Time frame: Preparation time: 10 minutes

Nutritional information (per serving):
- Calories: 120
- Total fat: 10g
- Saturated fat: 1.5g
- Sodium: 5mg
- Total carbohydrate: 8g
- Dietary fiber: 6g
- Sugars: 0.5g
- Protein: 2g

2. Classic Guacamole with Homemade Tortilla Chips:

Ingredients:
- 2 ripe avocados
- 1 tomato, diced
- 1/4 cup finely chopped onion
- 1/4 cup chopped fresh cilantro
- 1 lime, juiced
- Salt and pepper to taste
- Corn tortillas

Instructions:
1. In a bowl, mash the avocados until smooth.
2. Stir in the diced tomato, chopped onion, chopped cilantro, lime juice, salt, and pepper until well combined.

3. Preheat the oven to 350°F (175°C).
4. Cut the corn tortillas into triangles and place them on a baking sheet.
5. Bake for 8-10 minutes, or until crispy and golden brown.
6. Serve the guacamole with the homemade tortilla chips.

Time frame: Preparation time: 15 minutes; Cooking time: 8-10 minutes

Nutritional information (per serving, guacamole only):
- Calories: 90
- Total fat: 7g
- Saturated fat: 1g
- Sodium: 5mg
- Total carbohydrate: 7g
- Dietary fiber: 5g
- Sugars: 1g
- Protein: 1g

3. Spinach and Artichoke Dip with Whole Grain Pita Chips:

Ingredients:
- 1 cup frozen spinach, thawed and drained
- 1 cup canned artichoke hearts, drained and chopped
- 1/2 cup Greek yogurt
- 1/2 cup light cream cheese
- 1/4 cup grated Parmesan cheese
- 1/4 cup shredded mozzarella cheese
- 1 clove garlic, minced
- Salt and pepper to taste
- Whole grain pita bread, cut into triangles

Instructions:
1. Preheat the oven to 375°F (190°C).

2. In a mixing bowl, combine the thawed spinach, chopped artichoke hearts, Greek yogurt, cream cheese, Parmesan cheese, mozzarella cheese, minced garlic, salt, and pepper.

3. Transfer the mixture to a baking dish and spread it evenly.

4. Bake for 20-25 minutes, or until the dip is hot and bubbly.

5. While the dip is baking, cut the whole grain pita bread into triangles and arrange them on a baking sheet.

6. Bake the pita triangles for 8-10 minutes, or until crispy and lightly browned.

7. Serve the spinach and artichoke dip with the whole grain pita chips.

Time frame: Preparation time: 15 minutes; Cooking time: 20-25 minutes

Nutritional information (per serving, dip only):
- Calories: 110
- Total fat: 7g
- Saturated fat: 3.5g
- Sodium: 240mg
- Total carbohydrate: 6g
- Dietary fiber: 2g
- Sugars: 1g
- Protein: 7g

4. Roasted Red Pepper Hummus with Crudité:

Ingredients:
- 1 can (15 ounces) chickpeas, drained and rinsed
- 1/4 cup roasted red peppers
- 2 tablespoons tahini
- 2 tablespoons lemon juice
- 1 clove garlic, minced
- 1/2 teaspoon ground cumin

- Salt and pepper to taste
- Assorted fresh vegetables (carrots, celery, bell peppers, cucumber) for dipping

Instructions:
1. In a food processor, combine the chickpeas, roasted red peppers, tahini, lemon juice, minced garlic, ground cumin, salt, and pepper.
2. Process until smooth, scraping down the sides as needed.
3. If the hummus is too thick, add water, 1 tablespoon at a time, until desired consistency is reached.
4. Transfer the hummus to a serving bowl and garnish with a drizzle of olive oil and a sprinkle of paprika.
5. Serve with assorted fresh vegetables for dipping.

Time frame: Preparation time: 10 minutes

Nutritional information (per serving, hummus only):
- Calories: 70
- Total fat: 3g
- Saturated fat: 0g
- Sodium: 150mg
- Total carbohydrate: 9g
- Dietary fiber: 3g
- Sugars: 1g
- Protein: 3g

5. Tzatziki Dip with Cucumber Slices:

Ingredients:
- 1 cup Greek yogurt
- 1 cucumber, grated and squeezed to remove excess moisture
- 2 cloves garlic, minced

- 1 tablespoon fresh lemon juice
- 1 tablespoon chopped fresh dill
- Salt and pepper to taste
- Cucumber slices for dipping

Instructions:

1. In a bowl, combine the Greek yogurt, grated cucumber, minced garlic, lemon juice, chopped fresh dill, salt, and pepper.
2. Stir until well combined.
3. Refrigerate the tzatziki dip for at least 30 minutes to allow the flavors to meld.
4. Before serving, taste and adjust seasoning if needed.
5. Serve chilled with cucumber slices for dipping.

Time frame: Preparation time: 10 minutes; Chilling time: 30 minutes

Nutritional information (per serving, dip only):
- Calories: 40
- Total fat: 0g
- Saturated fat: 0g
- Sodium: 20mg
- Total carbohydrate: 5g
- Dietary fiber: 0g
- Sugars: 3g
- Protein: 5g

6. Black Bean Dip with Corn Tortilla Chips:

Ingredients:
- 1 can (15 ounces) black beans, drained and rinsed
- 1/4 cup salsa
- 1 tablespoon lime juice

- 1 teaspoon ground cumin
- 1/2 teaspoon chili powder
- Salt and pepper to taste
- Corn tortilla chips for dipping

Instructions:

1. In a food processor, combine the black beans, salsa, lime juice, ground cumin, chili powder, salt, and pepper.
2. Process until smooth, scraping down the sides as needed.
3. If the dip is too thick, add water, 1 tablespoon at a time, until desired consistency is reached.
4. Transfer the black bean dip to a serving bowl.
5. Serve with corn tortilla chips for dipping.

Time frame: Preparation time: 10 minutes

Nutritional information (per serving, dip only):
- Calories: 50
- Total fat: 0g
- Saturated fat: 0g
- Sodium: 200mg
- Total carbohydrate: 10g
- Dietary fiber: 4g
- Sugars: 1g
- Protein: 3g

7. Herbed Goat Cheese Spread with Crostini:

Ingredients:
- 4 ounces goat cheese, softened
- 2 tablespoons chopped fresh herbs (such as parsley, chives, and thyme)
- 1 tablespoon olive oil

- 1 teaspoon lemon zest
- Salt and pepper to taste
- Baguette, sliced and toasted

Instructions:

1. In a bowl, combine the softened goat cheese, chopped fresh herbs, olive oil, lemon zest, salt, and pepper.
2. Stir until the herbs are evenly distributed throughout the cheese.
3. Taste and adjust seasoning if needed.
4. Spread the herbed goat cheese mixture onto the toasted baguette slices.
5. Serve immediately as an appetizer or snack.

Time frame: Preparation time: 10 minutes

Nutritional information (per serving, spread only):
- Calories: 90
- Total fat: 7g
- Saturated fat: 4g
- Sodium: 110mg
- Total carbohydrate: 1g
- Dietary fiber: 0g
- Sugars: 0g
- Protein: 5g

8. Sun-Dried Tomato Tapenade with Crisp Breadsticks:

Ingredients:
- 1/2 cup sun-dried tomatoes (packed in oil), drained
- 2 tablespoons chopped Kalamata olives
- 1 tablespoon capers
- 1 clove garlic, minced
- 2 tablespoons chopped fresh basil

- 1 tablespoon lemon juice
- 2 tablespoons olive oil
- Salt and pepper to taste
- Breadsticks, for serving

Instructions:
1. In a food processor, combine the sun-dried tomatoes, chopped Kalamata olives, capers, minced garlic, chopped fresh basil, lemon juice, olive oil, salt, and pepper.
2. Pulse until the mixture forms a coarse paste, scraping down the sides as needed.
3. Taste and adjust seasoning if needed.
4. Transfer the sun-dried tomato tapenade to a serving bowl.
5. Serve with crisp breadsticks for dipping.

Time frame: Preparation time: 10 minutes

Nutritional information (per serving, tapenade only):
- Calories: 80
- Total fat: 7g
- Saturated fat: 1g
- Sodium: 200mg
- Total carbohydrate: 4g
- Dietary fiber: 1g
- Sugars: 2g
- Protein: 1g

9. Spicy Sriracha Dip with Rice Crackers:

Ingredients:
- 1/2 cup Greek yogurt
- 2 tablespoons Sriracha sauce

- 1 tablespoon honey
- 1 teaspoon lime juice
- 1/4 teaspoon garlic powder
- Salt to taste
- Rice crackers for dipping

Instructions:

1. In a bowl, whisk together the Greek yogurt, Sriracha sauce, honey, lime juice, garlic powder, and salt until well combined.
2. Taste the dip and adjust the seasoning as desired.
3. Serve the spicy Sriracha dip with rice crackers for dipping.

Time frame: Preparation time: 5 minutes

Nutritional information (per serving, dip only):
- Calories: 70
- Total fat: 0g
- Saturated fat: 0g
- Cholesterol: 0mg
- Sodium: 130mg
- Total carbohydrate: 15g
- Dietary fiber: 0g
- Sugars: 12g
- Protein: 2g

10. Mediterranean Olive Tapenade with Sliced Baguette:

Ingredients:
- 1 cup mixed olives (such as Kalamata and green olives), pitted
- 2 tablespoons capers
- 2 cloves garlic, minced
- 2 tablespoons chopped fresh parsley

- 2 tablespoons lemon juice
- 3 tablespoons olive oil
- Salt and pepper to taste
- Sliced baguette, for serving

Instructions:
1. In a food processor, combine the mixed olives, capers, minced garlic, chopped parsley, lemon juice, and olive oil.
2. Pulse the mixture until it reaches your desired consistency, scraping down the sides of the bowl as needed.
3. Season the tapenade with salt and pepper to taste, then pulse again to combine.
4. Transfer the tapenade to a serving bowl and drizzle with a little extra olive oil if desired.
5. Serve with sliced baguette for spreading.

Time frame: Preparation time: 10 minutes

Nutritional information (per serving, tapenade only):
- Calories: 70
- Total fat: 7g
- Saturated fat: 1g
- Cholesterol: 0mg
- Sodium: 320mg
- Total carbohydrate: 3g
- Dietary fiber: 2g
- Sugars: 0g
- Protein: 0g

CHAPTER 7

SWEET TREATS AND DESSERTS

Kidney-Friendly Dessert Swaps

1. Chia Seed Pudding Delight:

Ingredients:
- 1/4 cup chia seeds
- 1 cup unsweetened almond milk (or any milk of your choice)
- 1 tablespoon honey or maple syrup
- 1/2 teaspoon vanilla extract
- Fresh berries for topping

Instructions:
1. In a mixing bowl, combine chia seeds, almond milk, honey or maple syrup, and vanilla extract. Stir well to combine.
2. Let the mixture sit for 5 minutes, then stir again to prevent clumping.
3. Cover the bowl and refrigerate for at least 2 hours or overnight, until the mixture thickens into a pudding-like consistency.
4. Serve chilled, topped with fresh berries.

Cooking Time: 2 hours (including chilling time)
Nutritional Information (per serving):
- Calories: 120
- Protein: 4g
- Carbohydrates: 15g
- Fat: 6g
- Fiber: 8g

2. Avocado Chocolate Mousse:

Ingredients:
- 2 ripe avocados
- 1/4 cup unsweetened cocoa powder
- 1/4 cup honey or maple syrup
- 1 teaspoon vanilla extract
- Pinch of salt
- Fresh berries or chopped nuts for garnish (optional)

Instructions:
1. Scoop the flesh of the avocados into a blender or food processor.
2. Add cocoa powder, honey or maple syrup, vanilla extract, and a pinch of salt.
3. Blend until smooth and creamy, scraping down the sides as needed.
4. Divide the mousse into serving bowls and refrigerate for at least 1 hour to chill.
5. Garnish with fresh berries or chopped nuts before serving, if desired.

Cooking Time: 10 minutes (plus chilling time)
Nutritional Information (per serving):
- Calories: 200
- Protein: 3g
- Carbohydrates: 20g
- Fat: 15g
- Fiber: 8g

3. Coconut Flour Banana Bread:

Ingredients:
- 3 ripe bananas, mashed
- 3 eggs

- 1/4 cup coconut oil, melted
- 1/4 cup honey or maple syrup
- 1 teaspoon vanilla extract
- 3/4 cup coconut flour
- 1 teaspoon baking powder
- 1/2 teaspoon cinnamon
- Pinch of salt
- Optional: chopped walnuts or chocolate chips for topping

Instructions:
1. Preheat the oven to 350°F (175°C). Grease a loaf pan and set aside.
2. In a large mixing bowl, combine mashed bananas, eggs, melted coconut oil, honey or maple syrup, and vanilla extract. Mix well.
3. In a separate bowl, whisk together coconut flour, baking powder, cinnamon, and a pinch of salt.
4. Gradually add the dry ingredients to the wet ingredients, stirring until well combined and no lumps remain.
5. Pour the batter into the prepared loaf pan and smooth the top with a spatula. If desired, sprinkle chopped walnuts or chocolate chips on top.
6. Bake for 45-50 minutes, or until a toothpick inserted into the center comes out clean.
7. Allow the banana bread to cool in the pan for 10 minutes, then transfer to a wire rack to cool completely before slicing.

Cooking Time: 45-50 minutes
Nutritional Information (per serving, based on 12 servings):
- Calories: 150
- Protein: 3g
- Carbohydrates: 17g
- Fat: 8g
- Fiber: 4g

4. Baked Apples with Cinnamon Crumble:

Ingredients:
- 4 large apples, cored and halved
- 1 tablespoon lemon juice
- 1/2 teaspoon cinnamon
- 1/4 cup oats
- 2 tablespoons almond flour
- 1 tablespoon honey or maple syrup
- 1 tablespoon coconut oil, melted
- Pinch of salt

Instructions:
1. Preheat the oven to 350°F (175°C). Grease a baking dish and arrange the apple halves in a single layer.
2. Drizzle lemon juice over the apples and sprinkle with cinnamon.
3. In a small bowl, combine oats, almond flour, honey or maple syrup, melted coconut oil, and a pinch of salt. Mix until crumbly.
4. Spoon the crumble mixture evenly over the apple halves.
5. Bake for 25-30 minutes, or until the apples are tender and the crumble is golden brown.
6. Serve warm, optionally topped with a dollop of Greek yogurt or a sprinkle of chopped nuts.

Cooking Time: 25-30 minutes
Nutritional Information (per serving):
- Calories: 120
- Protein: 1g
- Carbohydrates: 22g
- Fat: 4g
- Fiber: 4g

5. Pumpkin Spice Oat Bars:

Ingredients:
- 2 cups rolled oats
- 1/2 cup pumpkin puree
- 1/4 cup honey or maple syrup
- 1/4 cup almond butter
- 1 teaspoon pumpkin pie spice
- 1/2 teaspoon vanilla extract
- Pinch of salt
- Optional: dark chocolate chips or dried fruit for topping

Instructions:
1. Preheat the oven to 350°F (175°C). Line an 8x8-inch baking dish with parchment paper, leaving some overhang on the sides.
2. In a large mixing bowl, combine rolled oats, pumpkin puree, honey or maple syrup, almond butter, pumpkin pie spice, vanilla extract, and a pinch of salt. Mix until well combined.
3. Press the mixture evenly into the prepared baking dish, using a spatula to smooth the top.
4. If desired, sprinkle dark chocolate chips or dried fruit on top and gently press them into the oat mixture.
5. Bake for 20-25 minutes, or until the edges are golden brown and the bars are set.
6. Allow the bars to cool in the pan for 10 minutes, then use the parchment paper to lift them out and transfer to a wire rack to cool completely before slicing into bars.

Cooking Time: 20-25 minutes
Nutritional Information (per serving, based on 12 servings):
- Calories: 130
- Protein: 3g

- Carbohydrates: 18g
- Fat: 5g
- Fiber: 3g

6. Almond Butter Energy Bites:

Ingredients:
- 1 cup rolled oats
- 1/2 cup almond butter
- 1/4 cup honey or maple syrup
- 1/4 cup unsweetened shredded coconut
- 2 tablespoons chia seeds
- 1 teaspoon vanilla extract
- Pinch of salt
- Optional: dark chocolate chips or chopped nuts for topping

Instructions:
1. In a mixing bowl, combine rolled oats, almond butter, honey or maple syrup, shredded coconut, chia seeds, vanilla extract, and a pinch of salt. Mix until well combined.
2. Roll the mixture into small balls, about 1 tablespoon each, and place them on a parchment-lined baking sheet.
3. If desired, press a dark chocolate chip or chopped nut into the top of each energy bite.
4. Refrigerate the energy bites for at least 30 minutes to firm up before serving.

Cooking Time: 30 minutes (including chilling time)
Nutritional Information (per serving, based on 12 servings):
- Calories: 120
- Protein: 3g
- Carbohydrates: 12g

- Fat: 7g
- Fiber: 2g

7. Lemon Poppy Seed Muffins (Low-Sodium):

Ingredients:
- 2 cups almond flour
- 1/4 cup coconut flour
- 1/4 cup honey or maple syrup
- 1/4 cup unsweetened applesauce
- 3 eggs
- 1/4 cup almond milk
- Zest and juice of 2 lemons
- 1 tablespoon poppy seeds
- 1 teaspoon baking powder
- 1/2 teaspoon vanilla extract
- Pinch of salt

Instructions:
1. Preheat the oven to 350°F (175°C). Line a muffin tin with paper liners or grease with coconut oil.
2. In a large mixing bowl, combine almond flour, coconut flour, honey or maple syrup, applesauce, eggs, almond milk, lemon zest and juice, poppy seeds, baking powder, vanilla extract, and a pinch of salt. Mix until well combined.
3. Divide the batter evenly among the muffin cups, filling each about 2/3 full.
4. Bake for 20-25 minutes, or until the muffins are golden brown and a toothpick inserted into the center comes out clean.
5. Allow the muffins to cool in the tin for 5 minutes, then transfer to a wire rack to cool completely before serving.

Cooking Time: 20-25 minutes

Nutritional Information (per muffin, based on 12 servings):
- Calories: 150
- Protein: 5g
- Carbohydrates: 12g
- Fat: 10g
- Fiber: 3g

8. Greek Yogurt Berry Parfait:

Ingredients:
- 1 cup Greek yogurt (unsweetened)
- 1 cup mixed berries (such as strawberries, blueberries, raspberries)
- 1/4 cup granola (low-sodium and low-phosphorus)
- 1 tablespoon honey or maple syrup (optional)

Instructions:
1. In a serving glass or bowl, layer Greek yogurt, mixed berries, and granola.
2. Repeat the layers until the glass or bowl is filled.
3. Drizzle honey or maple syrup on top, if desired, for extra sweetness.
4. Serve immediately, or refrigerate for up to 1 hour before serving to allow the flavors to meld.

Cooking Time: 5 minutes
Nutritional Information (per serving):
- Calories: 200
- Protein: 15g
- Carbohydrates: 25g
- Fat: 6g
- Fiber: 5g

9. Date and Walnut Truffles:

Ingredients:
- 1 cup pitted dates
- 1/2 cup walnuts
- 2 tablespoons unsweetened cocoa powder
- 1 teaspoon vanilla extract
- Pinch of salt
- Unsweetened shredded coconut for rolling (optional)

Instructions:
1. In a food processor, combine pitted dates, walnuts, cocoa powder, vanilla extract, and a pinch of salt.
2. Pulse until the mixture comes together and forms a sticky dough.
3. Roll the dough into small balls, about 1 tablespoon each.
4. If desired, roll the truffles in unsweetened shredded coconut for added texture and flavor.
5. Refrigerate the truffles for at least 30 minutes before serving.

Cooking Time: 30 minutes (including chilling time)
Nutritional Information (per serving, based on 12 servings):
- Calories: 100
- Protein: 2g
- Carbohydrates: 15g
- Fat: 5g
- Fiber: 2g

10. Carrot Cake Protein Bites:

Ingredients:
- 1 cup rolled oats
- 1/2 cup shredded carrots
- 1/4 cup almond butter
- 1/4 cup honey or maple syrup

- 1/4 cup chopped walnuts
- 1 teaspoon cinnamon
- 1/2 teaspoon vanilla extract
- Pinch of salt
- Unsweetened shredded coconut for rolling (optional)

Instructions:

1. In a mixing bowl, combine rolled oats, shredded carrots, almond butter, honey or maple syrup, chopped walnuts, cinnamon, vanilla extract, and a pinch of salt. Mix until well combined.
2. Roll the mixture into small balls, about 1 tablespoon each.
3. If desired, roll the balls in unsweetened shredded coconut for added flavor and texture.
4. Refrigerate the protein bites for at least 30 minutes before serving.

Cooking Time: 30 minutes (including chilling time)
Nutritional Information (per serving, based on 12 servings):
- Calories: 120
- Protein: 3g
- Carbohydrates: 15g
- Fat: 6g
- Fiber: 2g

These recipes offer delicious and nutritious options for satisfying your sweet cravings while adhering to kidney-friendly dietary guidelines. Enjoy these treats as part of a balanced diet to support your kidney health and overall well-being.

Fruit-Based Desserts for Seniors

Below are the revised recipes with corrected ingredients and measurements, clear instructions, appropriate time frames, and nutritional information where available:

1. Grilled Pineapple with Honey and Mint:
Ingredients:
- 1 pineapple, peeled and cored, cut into rings
- 2 tablespoons honey
- 1 tablespoon fresh mint leaves, chopped

Instructions:
1. Preheat the grill to medium-high heat.
2. Brush each pineapple ring with honey on both sides.
3. Grill the pineapple rings for 2-3 minutes per side, until grill marks appear.
4. Remove from the grill and sprinkle with chopped mint leaves.
5. Serve warm as a refreshing dessert.

Nutritional Information (per serving):
- Calories: 110
- Protein: 1g
- Fat: 0g
- Carbohydrates: 28g
- Fiber: 3g
- Sugar: 20g

2. Berry Coconut Ice Pops:
Ingredients:
- 1 cup mixed berries (strawberries, blueberries, raspberries)
- 1 cup coconut water
- 2 tablespoons honey or maple syrup

Instructions:
1. In a blender, combine mixed berries, coconut water, and honey or maple syrup.
2. Blend until smooth.

3. Pour the mixture into ice pop molds.

4. Insert sticks and freeze for at least 4 hours, or until firm.

5. To unmold, run warm water over the molds briefly.

Nutritional Information (per serving):

- Calories: 50

- Protein: 0g

- Fat: 0g

- Carbohydrates: 13g

- Fiber: 2g

- Sugar: 9g

3. Mango Salsa with Cinnamon Tortilla Chips:

Ingredients for Salsa:

- 2 ripe mangoes, peeled and diced

- 1/2 red onion, finely chopped

- 1 jalapeño pepper, seeded and minced

- 1/4 cup fresh cilantro, chopped

- Juice of 1 lime

- Salt to taste

Ingredients for Cinnamon Tortilla Chips:

- 4 whole wheat tortillas

- 1 tablespoon olive oil

- 1 tablespoon honey

- 1 teaspoon ground cinnamon

Instructions:

1. In a bowl, combine diced mangoes, red onion, jalapeño pepper, cilantro, lime juice, and salt. Mix well and set aside.

2. Preheat the oven to 350°F (175°C).

3. Brush both sides of tortillas with olive oil.

4. Cut tortillas into wedges and place on a baking sheet.

5. In a small bowl, mix honey and cinnamon. Brush mixture over tortilla wedges.

6. Bake for 10-12 minutes or until crisp.

7. Serve cinnamon tortilla chips with mango salsa.

Nutritional Information (per serving - salsa only):
- Calories: 60
- Protein: 1g
- Fat: 0g
- Carbohydrates: 15g
- Fiber: 2g
- Sugar: 11g

4. Poached Pears with Vanilla Yogurt Drizzle:
Ingredients:
- 4 ripe pears, peeled and cored
- 2 cups water
- 1/2 cup honey or maple syrup
- 1 teaspoon vanilla extract
- 1 cup plain Greek yogurt

Instructions:
1. In a saucepan, combine water, honey or maple syrup, and vanilla extract. Bring to a simmer.

2. Add pears to the saucepan and simmer for 15-20 minutes, or until pears are tender.

3. Remove pears from the poaching liquid and let cool slightly.

4. In a small bowl, mix Greek yogurt with a splash of vanilla extract.

5. Drizzle vanilla yogurt over poached pears before serving.

Nutritional Information (per serving):

- Calories: 180
- Protein: 6g
- Fat: 0g
- Carbohydrates: 40g
- Fiber: 4g
- Sugar: 28g

5. Strawberry Kiwi Sorbet:

Ingredients:
- 2 cups strawberries, hulled
- 2 kiwis, peeled and sliced
- 1/4 cup honey or maple syrup
- Juice of 1 lemon

Instructions:
1. In a blender, combine strawberries, kiwis, honey or maple syrup, and lemon juice.
2. Blend until smooth.
3. Pour the mixture into a shallow dish and freeze for 4-6 hours, stirring occasionally.
4. Once frozen, blend again until smooth and creamy.
5. Serve immediately as a refreshing dessert.

Nutritional Information (per serving):
- Calories: 90
- Protein: 1g
- Fat: 0g
- Carbohydrates: 23g
- Fiber: 3g
- Sugar: 18g

6. Peach and Blueberry Cobbler:

Ingredients:
- 4 peaches, peeled and sliced
- 1 cup blueberries
- 1 tablespoon lemon juice
- 1/4 cup honey or maple syrup
- 1 cup oats
- 1/4 cup whole wheat flour
- 1/4 cup almond flour
- 1/4 cup coconut oil, melted
- 1 teaspoon vanilla extract
- 1 teaspoon ground cinnamon

Instructions:
1. Preheat the oven to 350°F (175°C).
2. In a mixing bowl, combine sliced peaches, blueberries, lemon juice, and honey or maple syrup. Mix well and transfer to a baking dish.
3. In another bowl, combine oats, whole wheat flour, almond flour, melted coconut oil, vanilla extract, and ground cinnamon. Mix until crumbly.
4. Spread the oat mixture evenly over the fruit in the baking dish.
5. Bake for 30-35 minutes, or until the topping is golden brown and the fruit is bubbling.
6. Serve warm with a dollop of Greek yogurt or a scoop of vanilla ice cream, if desired.

Nutritional Information (per serving):
- Calories: 220
- Protein: 4g
- Fat: 8g
- Carbohydrates: 38g
- Fiber: 5g
- Sugar: 21g

7. Baked Cinnamon Apples:
Ingredients:
- 4 apples, cored and sliced
- 1 tablespoon lemon juice
- 1 tablespoon honey or maple syrup
- 1 teaspoon ground cinnamon

Instructions:
1. Preheat the oven to 350°F (175°C).
2. In a bowl, toss sliced apples with lemon juice, honey or maple syrup, and ground cinnamon until evenly coated.
3. Spread the apples in a single layer on a baking sheet lined with parchment paper.
4. Bake for 20-25 minutes, or until apples are tender and lightly caramelized.
5. Serve warm as a comforting dessert or snack.

Nutritional Information (per serving):
- Calories: 90
- Protein: 0g
- Fat: 0g
- Carbohydrates: 24g
- Fiber: 4g
- Sugar: 18g

8. Watermelon Lime Granita:
Ingredients:
- 4 cups seedless watermelon, cubed
- Juice of 2 limes
- 2 tablespoons honey or maple syrup
- Zest of 1 lime (optional)
- Mint leaves, for garnish

Instructions:

1. In a blender, combine watermelon cubes, lime juice, honey or maple syrup, and lime zest (if using).

2. Blend until smooth.

3. Pour the mixture into a shallow dish and freeze for 2-3 hours, stirring occasionally with a fork to break up ice crystals.

4. Once frozen, scrape the granita with a fork to create a fluffy texture.

5. Serve immediately in chilled glasses, garnished with fresh mint leaves.

Nutritional Information (per serving):

- Calories: 80
- Protein: 1g
- Fat: 0g
- Carbohydrates: 20g
- Fiber: 1g
- Sugar: 17g

9. Kiwi and Banana Smoothie Bowl:

Ingredients:

- 2 ripe kiwis, peeled and sliced
- 2 ripe bananas, peeled and sliced
- 1/2 cup plain Greek yogurt
- 1/4 cup almond milk
- 1 tablespoon honey or maple syrup
- Toppings of choice (granola, sliced almonds, chia seeds, shredded coconut)

Instructions:

1. In a blender, combine kiwis, bananas, Greek yogurt, almond milk, and honey or maple syrup.

2. Blend until smooth and creamy.

3. Pour the smoothie into bowls.

4. Top with your favorite toppings, such as granola, sliced almonds, chia seeds, and shredded coconut.

5. Serve immediately for a nutritious and satisfying breakfast or snack.

Nutritional Information (per serving):
- Calories: 180
- Protein: 6g
- Fat: 2g
- Carbohydrates: 35g
- Fiber: 6g
- Sugar: 21g

10. Citrus Fruit Salad with Honey-Lime Dressing:
Ingredients:
- 2 oranges, peeled and segmented
- 2 grapefruits, peeled and segmented
- 2 kiwis, peeled and sliced
- 1 tablespoon honey
- Juice of 1 lime
- Fresh mint leaves, for garnish

Instructions:
1. In a large bowl, combine orange segments, grapefruit segments, and sliced kiwis.
2. In a small bowl, whisk together honey and lime juice to make the dressing.
3. Drizzle the honey-lime dressing over the fruit salad and toss gently to coat.
4. Garnish with fresh mint leaves before serving.

Nutritional Information (per serving):
- Calories: 110
- Protein: 2g
- Fat: 0g

- Carbohydrates: 28g
- Fiber: 5g
- Sugar: 20g

Decadent but Healthy Indulgences

1. Dark Chocolate Covered Almonds

Ingredients:
- 1 cup raw almonds
- 4 ounces dark chocolate (70% cocoa or higher)
- Optional: sea salt flakes for garnish

Instructions:
1. Line a baking sheet with parchment paper.
2. In a microwave-safe bowl, melt the dark chocolate in 30-second intervals, stirring in between until smooth.
3. Add the almonds to the melted chocolate, stirring until they are evenly coated.
4. Using a fork, remove the almonds from the chocolate one by one, allowing excess chocolate to drip off, and place them on the prepared baking sheet.
5. Sprinkle sea salt flakes over the almonds if desired.
6. Allow the chocolate-covered almonds to set at room temperature for about 1 hour or until the chocolate hardens.
7. Once set, store the dark chocolate-covered almonds in an airtight container at room temperature for up to 1 week.

Nutritional Information (per serving - 1 ounce):
- Calories: 160
- Total Fat: 12g
- Saturated Fat: 3g
- Carbohydrates: 9g

- Fiber: 3g
- Sugar: 3g
- Protein: 5g

Time frame: Approximately 1 hour.

2. Peanut Butter Banana Ice Cream

Ingredients:
- 3 ripe bananas, sliced and frozen
- 2 tablespoons natural peanut butter
- Optional toppings: chopped peanuts, dark chocolate chips

Instructions:
1. In a food processor or high-speed blender, add the frozen banana slices and peanut butter.
2. Blend until smooth and creamy, scraping down the sides of the bowl as needed.
3. Serve immediately as soft-serve ice cream or transfer to a container and freeze for 1-2 hours for a firmer texture.
4. If desired, sprinkle with chopped peanuts or dark chocolate chips before serving.

Nutritional Information (per serving - 1/2 cup):
- Calories: 150
- Total Fat: 6g
- Saturated Fat: 1g
- Carbohydrates: 23g
- Fiber: 3g
- Sugar: 12g
- Protein: 3g

Time frame: Approximately 10 minutes, plus freezing time.

3. Quinoa Chocolate Chip Cookies

Ingredients:
- 1 cup cooked quinoa, cooled
- 1/2 cup almond flour
- 1/4 cup coconut sugar
- 1/4 cup maple syrup
- 1/4 cup coconut oil, melted
- 1 teaspoon vanilla extract
- 1/2 teaspoon baking powder
- 1/4 teaspoon salt
- 1/2 cup dark chocolate chips

Instructions:
1. Preheat your oven to 350°F (175°C). Line a baking sheet with parchment paper.
2. In a large mixing bowl, combine cooked quinoa, almond flour, coconut sugar, maple syrup, melted coconut oil, vanilla extract, baking powder, and salt. Mix until well combined.
3. Fold in the dark chocolate chips until evenly distributed throughout the dough.
4. Scoop tablespoon-sized portions of dough and roll them into balls. Place them on the prepared baking sheet, leaving space between each cookie.
5. Flatten each cookie slightly with the palm of your hand.
6. Bake in the preheated oven for 12-15 minutes, or until the edges are golden brown.
7. Remove from the oven and let the cookies cool on the baking sheet for 5 minutes before transferring them to a wire rack to cool completely.
8. Store the quinoa chocolate chip cookies in an airtight container at room temperature for up to 5 days.

Nutritional Information (per cookie):
- Calories: 120
- Total Fat: 7g
- Saturated Fat: 4g
- Carbohydrates: 13g
- Fiber: 1g
- Sugar: 7g
- Protein: 2g

Time frame: Approximately 30 minutes.

4. Greek Yogurt Cheesecake Bites

Ingredients:
- 1 cup plain Greek yogurt
- 1/4 cup honey or maple syrup
- 1 teaspoon vanilla extract
- Zest of 1 lemon
- Graham cracker crumbs (optional, for coating)

Instructions:
1. In a mixing bowl, combine Greek yogurt, honey or maple syrup, vanilla extract, and lemon zest. Mix until smooth and well combined.
2. Line a mini muffin tin with paper liners.
3. Spoon the yogurt mixture into the mini muffin tin, filling each cup about halfway.
4. Place the muffin tin in the freezer and freeze for 2-3 hours, or until the yogurt mixture is firm.
5. Once firm, remove the cheesecake bites from the muffin tin and, if desired, roll them in graham cracker crumbs to coat.

6. Serve immediately or transfer to an airtight container and store in the freezer for up to 1 week.

Nutritional Information (per bite):
- Calories: 30
- Total Fat: 0g
- Saturated Fat: 0g
- Carbohydrates: 4g
- Fiber: 0g
- Sugar: 4g
- Protein: 3g

Time frame: Approximately 10 minutes, plus freezing time.

5. Chocolate Avocado Truffles

Ingredients:
- 2 ripe avocados
- 1/4 cup unsweetened cocoa powder
- 1/4 cup honey or maple syrup
- 1 teaspoon vanilla extract
- Pinch of salt
- Unsweetened cocoa powder, shredded coconut, or crushed nuts for coating (optional)

Instructions:
1. Cut the avocados in half, remove the pits, and scoop the flesh into a bowl.
2. Add cocoa powder, honey or maple syrup, vanilla extract, and salt to the bowl with the avocado.
3. Mash and stir the ingredients together until smooth and well combined.
4. Cover the bowl with plastic wrap and refrigerate the mixture for 30 minutes to 1 hour to firm up.

5. Once chilled, scoop tablespoon-sized portions of the mixture and roll them into balls.

6. Roll the truffles in unsweetened cocoa powder, shredded coconut, or crushed nuts for coating, if desired.

7. Place the coated truffles on a plate or baking sheet lined with parchment paper.

8. Chill the truffles in the refrigerator for another 30 minutes before serving.

9. Store the chocolate avocado truffles in an airtight container in the refrigerator for up to 3 days.

Nutritional Information (per truffle):
- Calories: 60
- Total Fat: 4g
- Saturated Fat: 1g
- Carbohydrates: 7g
- Fiber: 2g
- Sugar: 4g
- Protein: 1g

Time frame: Approximately 1 hour, including chilling time.

6. Coconut Macaroons with Dark Chocolate Drizzle

Ingredients:
- 2 cups unsweetened shredded coconut
- 1/4 cup honey or maple syrup
- 2 egg whites
- 1 teaspoon vanilla extract
- 4 ounces dark chocolate, melted

Instructions:

1. Preheat your oven to 325°F (160°C). Line a baking sheet with parchment paper.

2. In a mixing bowl, combine shredded coconut, honey or maple syrup, egg whites, and vanilla extract. Mix until well combined.

3. Use a spoon or cookie scoop to form the mixture into small mounds and place them on the prepared baking sheet.

4. Bake in the preheated oven for 20-25 minutes, or until the edges of the macaroons are golden brown.

5. Remove from the oven and let the macaroons cool on the baking sheet for 5 minutes before transferring them to a wire rack to cool completely.

6. Once the macaroons are cooled, drizzle melted dark chocolate over the top of each macaroon.

7. Allow the chocolate to set at room temperature or place the macaroons in the refrigerator for 10-15 minutes to speed up the process.

8. Store the coconut macaroons in an airtight container at room temperature for up to 5 days.

Nutritional Information (per macaroon):
- Calories: 80
- Total Fat: 5g
- Saturated Fat: 4g
- Carbohydrates: 8g
- Fiber: 2g
- Sugar: 6g
- Protein: 1g

Time frame: Approximately 40 minutes.

7. Pistachio Cranberry Bark

Ingredients:
- 8 ounces dark chocolate, chopped

- 1/4 cup dried cranberries
- 1/4 cup shelled pistachios, chopped
- Sea salt flakes (optional)

Instructions:
1. Line a baking sheet with parchment paper.
2. In a heatproof bowl set over a pot of simmering water (double boiler), melt the dark chocolate, stirring occasionally until smooth.
3. Once melted, pour the chocolate onto the prepared baking sheet and spread it into an even layer using a spatula.
4. Sprinkle the dried cranberries and chopped pistachios evenly over the melted chocolate.
5. If desired, sprinkle a pinch of sea salt flakes over the bark.
6. Place the baking sheet in the refrigerator for 1-2 hours, or until the chocolate is firm.
7. Once set, break the bark into pieces and store it in an airtight container in the refrigerator for up to 1 week.

Nutritional Information (per serving - 1 ounce):
- Calories: 120
- Total Fat: 8g
- Saturated Fat: 4g
- Carbohydrates: 12g
- Fiber: 2g
- Sugar: 8g
- Protein: 2g

Time frame: Approximately 2 hours, including chilling time.

8. Maple Roasted Pecans

Ingredients:

- 2 cups pecan halves
- 2 tablespoons pure maple syrup
- 1/2 teaspoon ground cinnamon
- Pinch of salt

Instructions:

1. Preheat your oven to 350°F (175°C). Line a baking sheet with parchment paper.
2. In a mixing bowl, combine pecan halves, maple syrup, ground cinnamon, and a pinch of salt. Toss until the pecans are evenly coated.
3. Spread the pecans in a single layer on the prepared baking sheet.
4. Bake in the preheated oven for 10-12 minutes, stirring halfway through, until the pecans are fragrant and lightly toasted.
5. Remove from the oven and let the pecans cool completely on the baking sheet.
6. Once cooled, transfer the maple roasted pecans to an airtight container and store them at room temperature for up to 1 week.

Nutritional Information (per serving - 1 ounce):
- Calories: 160
- Total Fat: 16g
- Saturated Fat: 1g
- Carbohydrates: 4g
- Fiber: 2g
- Sugar: 2g
- Protein: 2g

Time frame: Approximately 20 minutes.

9. Hazelnut Chocolate Spread Stuffed Dates

Ingredients:

- 12 Medjool dates, pitted
- 1/4 cup hazelnut chocolate spread (check for kidney-friendly options)
- Optional toppings: chopped hazelnuts, shredded coconut

Instructions:

1. Using a small knife, make a lengthwise slit in each date and remove the pit.

2. Fill each date with hazelnut chocolate spread, using about 1 teaspoon for each date.

3. If desired, roll the stuffed dates in chopped hazelnuts or shredded coconut for additional flavor and texture.

4. Arrange the stuffed dates on a serving platter and serve immediately, or store them in an airtight container in the refrigerator for up to 3 days.

Nutritional Information (per date):
- Calories: 90
- Total Fat: 2g
- Saturated Fat: 0g
- Carbohydrates: 18g
- Fiber: 2g
- Sugar: 16g
- Protein: 1g

Time frame: Approximately 10 minutes.

10. Almond Flour Chocolate Brownies

Ingredients:
- 1 cup almond flour
- 1/4 cup unsweetened cocoa powder
- 1/4 teaspoon baking soda
- 1/4 teaspoon salt

- 1/4 cup honey or maple syrup
- 1/4 cup coconut oil, melted
- 2 eggs
- 1 teaspoon vanilla extract
- 1/4 cup dark chocolate chips

Instructions:

1. Preheat your oven to 350°F (175°C). Grease or line an 8x8-inch baking pan with parchment paper.

2. In a mixing bowl, whisk together almond flour, cocoa powder, baking soda, and salt.

3. In a separate bowl, combine honey or maple syrup, melted coconut oil, eggs, and vanilla extract. Mix until well combined.

4. Add the wet ingredients to the dry ingredients and mix until smooth.

5. Fold in the dark chocolate chips.

6. Pour the batter into the prepared baking pan and spread it into an even layer.

7. Bake in the preheated oven for 20-25 minutes, or until a toothpick inserted into the center comes out clean.

8. Remove from the oven and let the brownies cool completely in the pan before slicing and serving.

9. Store the almond flour chocolate brownies in an airtight container at room temperature for up to 3 days.

Nutritional Information (per brownie - 1/16th of the pan):

- Calories: 120
- Total Fat: 9g
- Saturated Fat: 4g
- Carbohydrates: 9g
- Fiber: 1g
- Sugar: 6g
- Protein: 3g

Time frame: Approximately 30 minutes.

BONUS 30-DAYS MEAL PLAN

Week 1:

Day 1:
- Breakfast: Greek Yogurt Parfait with Fresh Berries and Almonds
- Lunch: Mediterranean Chickpea Salad with Feta and Cucumber
- Dinner: Herb-Crusted Baked Salmon with Lemon-Dill Sauce, served with Garlic Roasted Brussels Sprouts
- Snack: Nutty Energy Bites

Day 2:
- Breakfast: Spinach and Feta Omelette Roll-Ups
- Lunch: Garden Harvest Minestrone
- Dinner: Quinoa Stuffed Bell Peppers
- Snack: Veggie Sticks with Hummus

Day 3:
- Breakfast: Banana Nut Overnight Oats
- Lunch: Creamy Mushroom and Wild Rice Soup
- Dinner: Lemon Herb Grilled Chicken Breast with Quinoa Pilaf with Herbs and Lemon
- Snack: Cheese and Whole Grain Crackers

Day 4:
- Breakfast: Quinoa Breakfast Bowl with Roasted Vegetables
- Lunch: Asian-Inspired Sesame Ginger Noodle Salad
- Dinner: Lentil and Vegetable Shepherd's Pie
- Snack: Mini Quiches with Spinach and Feta

Day 5:
- Breakfast: Smoked Salmon and Avocado Toast
- Lunch: Coconut Curry Lentil Soup
- Dinner: Garlic Butter Baked Salmon, served with Lemon-Glazed Green Beans
- Snack: Apple Slices with Almond Butter

Day 6:
- Breakfast: Berry Blast Smoothie with Spinach and Flaxseed
- Lunch: Roasted Tomato Basil Bisque with Grilled Cheese Sandwiches using Whole Grain Bread
- Dinner: Spicy Cajun Blackened Tilapia with Wild Rice with Mushrooms and Herbs
- Snack: Chia Seed Pudding with Mango and Coconut

Day 7:
- Breakfast: Sweet Potato and Black Bean Hash
- Lunch: Greek Orzo Pasta Salad with Cherry Tomatoes and Cucumber
- Dinner: Mediterranean Chicken Skewers with Tzatziki Sauce, served with Mediterranean Chickpea Salad
- Snack: Greek Yogurt Parfait Cups

Day 8:
- Breakfast: Turkey Sausage and Egg Breakfast Sandwich
- Lunch: Lemon Chicken Orzo Soup with a side of Spinach and Feta Stuffed Portobello Mushrooms
- Dinner: Rosemary Roasted Turkey Breast with Mediterranean Quinoa Salad with Feta and Olives
- Snack: Trail Mix Popcorn Balls

Day 9:
- Breakfast: Kiwi Strawberry Kale Smoothie

- Lunch: Butternut Squash and Apple Soup with Avocado and Tomato Bruschetta on Whole Grain Toast
- Dinner: Honey Mustard Glazed Turkey Meatballs with Lentil and Brown Rice Casserole
- Snack: Protein-Packed Deviled Eggs

Day 10:
- Breakfast: Quinoa Breakfast Bowl with Roasted Vegetables
- Lunch: Spicy Black Bean and Sweet Potato Soup with a side of Caprese Salad Skewers with Basil Pesto Drizzle
- Dinner: Sesame Ginger Glazed Mahi-Mahi with Mediterranean Chickpea Salad
- Snack: Banana-Oatmeal Muffins

Day 11:
- Breakfast: Greek Yogurt Parfait with Fresh Berries and Almonds
- Lunch: Creamy Mushroom and Wild Rice Soup with Grilled Turkey and Swiss Cheese Wraps with Whole Grain Tortillas
- Dinner: Garlic Herb Grilled Chicken Breast with Quinoa Pilaf with Herbs and Lemon
- Snack: Greek Yogurt Cheesecake Bites

Day 12:
- Breakfast: Spinach and Feta Omelette Roll-Ups
- Lunch: Moroccan Chickpea Stew with Greek Orzo Pasta Salad with Cherry Tomatoes and Cucumber
- Dinner: Mediterranean Chicken Skewers with Tzatziki Sauce, served with Mediterranean Quinoa Salad with Feta and Olives
- Snack: Apple Slices with Almond Butter

Day 13:
- Breakfast: Berry Blast Smoothie with Spinach and Flaxseed

- Lunch: Thai Coconut Chicken Soup with a side of Grilled Peach and Arugula Salad with Balsamic Glaze
- Dinner: Herb-Crusted Baked Cod Fillets with Coconut Lime Grilled Shrimp Skewers
- Snack: Nutty Energy Bites

Day 14:
- Breakfast: Sweet Potato and Black Bean Hash
- Lunch: Greek Orzo Pasta Salad with Cherry Tomatoes and Cucumber with Stuffed Mushrooms with Creamy Herb Filling
- Dinner: Lemon Herb Grilled Chicken Breast with Quinoa Pilaf with Herbs and Lemon
- Snack: Cheese and Whole Grain Crackers

Week 3:

Day 15:
- Breakfast: Banana Nut Overnight Oats
- Lunch: Coconut Curry Lentil Soup with Mediterranean Quinoa Salad with Feta and Olives
- Dinner: Herb-Crusted Baked Salmon with Lemon-Dill Sauce, served with Garlic Roasted Brussels Sprouts
- Snack: Trail Mix Popcorn Balls

Day 16:
- Breakfast: Quinoa Breakfast Bowl with Roasted Vegetables
- Lunch: Asian-Inspired Sesame Ginger Noodle Salad with Avocado and Tomato Bruschetta on Whole Grain Toast
- Dinner: Spicy Cajun Blackened Tilapia with Wild Rice with Mushrooms and Herbs
- Snack: Protein-Packed Deviled Eggs

Day 17:
- Breakfast: Greek Yogurt Parfait with Fresh Berries and Almonds
- Lunch: Lemon Chicken Orzo Soup with Spinach and Feta Stuffed Portobello Mushrooms
- Dinner: Rosemary Roasted Turkey Breast with Mediterranean Chickpea Salad with Feta and Olives
- Snack: Banana-Oatmeal Muffins

Day 18:
- Breakfast: Kiwi Strawberry Kale Smoothie
- Lunch: Butternut Squash and Apple Soup with Turkey and Vegetable Breakfast Casserole
- Dinner: Honey Mustard Glazed Turkey Meatballs with Lentil and Brown Rice Casserole
- Snack: Greek Yogurt Cheesecake Bites

Day 19:
- Breakfast: Quinoa Breakfast Bowl with Roasted Vegetables
- Lunch: Spicy Black Bean and Sweet Potato Soup with Caprese Salad Skewers with Basil Pesto Drizzle
- Dinner: Sesame Ginger Glazed Mahi-Mahi with Mediterranean Chickpea Salad
- Snack: Apple Slices with Almond Butter

Day 20:
- Breakfast: Greek Yogurt Parfait with Fresh Berries and Almonds
- Lunch: Creamy Mushroom and Wild Rice Soup with Grilled Turkey and Swiss Cheese Wraps with Whole Grain Tortillas
- Dinner: Garlic Herb Grilled Chicken Breast with Quinoa Pilaf with Herbs and Lemon
- Snack: Nutty Energy Bites

Day 21:
- Breakfast: Berry Blast Smoothie with Spinach and Flaxseed
- Lunch: Thai Coconut Chicken Soup with Grilled Peach and Arugula Salad with Balsamic Glaze
- Dinner: Herb-Crusted Baked Cod Fillets with Coconut Lime Grilled Shrimp Skewers
- Snack: Cheese and Whole Grain Crackers

Week 4:

Day 22:
- Breakfast: Spinach and Feta Omelette Roll-Ups
- Lunch: Mediterranean Chickpea Salad with Feta and Cucumber
- Dinner: Herb-Crusted Baked Salmon with Lemon-Dill Sauce, served with Garlic Roasted Brussels Sprouts
- Snack: Nutty Energy Bites

Day 23:
- Breakfast: Banana Nut Overnight Oats
- Lunch: Coconut Curry Lentil Soup with Mediterranean Quinoa Salad with Feta and Olives
- Dinner: Rosemary Roasted Turkey Breast with Mediterranean Chickpea Salad with Feta and Olives
- Snack: Greek Yogurt Parfait Cups

Day 24:
- Breakfast: Greek Yogurt Parfait with Fresh Berries and Almonds
- Lunch: Lemon Chicken Orzo Soup with Spinach and Feta Stuffed Portobello Mushrooms
- Dinner: Garlic Butter Baked Salmon with Lemon-Glazed Green Beans
- Snack: Trail Mix Popcorn Balls

Day 25:
- Breakfast: Quinoa Breakfast Bowl with Roasted Vegetables
- Lunch: Asian-Inspired Sesame Ginger Noodle Salad with Avocado and Tomato Bruschetta on Whole Grain Toast
- Dinner: Honey Mustard Glazed Turkey Meatballs with Lentil and Brown Rice Casserole
- Snack: Banana-Oatmeal Muffins

Day 26:
- Breakfast: Smoked Salmon and Avocado Toast
- Lunch: Butternut Squash and Apple Soup with Turkey and Vegetable Breakfast Casserole
- Dinner: Sesame Ginger Glazed Mahi-Mahi with Mediterranean Chickpea Salad with Feta and Olives
- Snack: Protein-Packed Deviled Eggs

Day 27:
- Breakfast: Berry Blast Smoothie with Spinach and Flaxseed
- Lunch: Spicy Black Bean and Sweet Potato Soup with Caprese Salad Skewers with Basil Pesto Drizzle
- Dinner: Grilled Pineapple with Honey and Mint
- Snack: Apple Slices with Almond Butter

Day 28:
- Breakfast: Greek Yogurt Parfait with Fresh Berries and Almonds
- Lunch: Creamy Mushroom and Wild Rice Soup with Grilled Turkey and Swiss Cheese Wraps with Whole Grain Tortillas
- Dinner: Lemon Herb Grilled Chicken Breast with Quinoa Pilaf with Herbs and Lemon
- Snack: Greek Yogurt Cheesecake Bites

Day 29:
- Breakfast: Sweet Potato and Black Bean Hash
- Lunch: Thai Coconut Chicken Soup with Grilled Peach and Arugula Salad with Balsamic Glaze
- Dinner: Herb-Crusted Baked Cod Fillets with Coconut Lime Grilled Shrimp Skewers
- Snack: Cheese and Whole Grain Crackers

Day 30:
- Breakfast: Quinoa Breakfast Bowl with Roasted Vegetables
- Lunch: Greek Orzo Pasta Salad with Cherry Tomatoes and Cucumber with Stuffed Mushrooms with Creamy Herb Filling
- Dinner: Mediterranean Chicken Skewers with Tzatziki Sauce, served with Mediterranean Quinoa Salad with Feta and Olives
- Snack: Apple Slices with Almond Butter

CHAPTER 8

BEVERAGES AND HYDRATION TIPS

It's crucial to emphasize the importance of proper hydration and beverage choices for seniors, particularly those managing stage 3 kidney disease. Hydration plays a vital role in kidney function and overall health, as adequate fluid intake helps to flush out toxins and waste products from the body while maintaining electrolyte balance. However, for seniors with kidney disease, certain considerations must be made when selecting beverages to prevent exacerbating symptoms and supporting optimal kidney function.

Refreshing Drink Options

1. Water: Undoubtedly, water is the best choice for hydration. It's calorie-free, readily available, and essential for maintaining fluid balance in the body. Encourage seniors to drink water throughout the day, aiming for at least 8-10 cups daily, unless otherwise restricted by their healthcare provider.

2. Herbal Teas: Herbal teas such as chamomile, peppermint, and ginger can be soothing and hydrating alternatives to plain water. These teas are naturally caffeine-free and offer additional health benefits, such as aiding digestion and reducing inflammation.

3. Infused Water: Add flavor to plain water by infusing it with slices of citrus fruits, berries, cucumber, or mint leaves. Infused water provides a refreshing taste without added sugars or calories, making it an excellent choice for seniors watching their sugar intake.

4. Coconut Water: Low in potassium and naturally hydrating, coconut water is a good option for seniors with kidney disease. It contains electrolytes such as potassium and sodium, which can help replenish lost fluids and maintain hydration levels, especially after physical activity.

5. Homemade Smoothies: Blend together fruits such as berries, apples, and bananas with water or low-potassium milk alternatives (e.g., almond milk or rice milk) to create delicious and hydrating smoothies. Avoid adding high-potassium fruits like oranges, kiwis, and mangoes in large quantities.

Hydration Strategies for Seniors

1. Drink Regularly Throughout the Day: Encourage seniors to sip fluids regularly rather than waiting until they feel thirsty. Set reminders or provide easily accessible water bottles to promote consistent hydration.

2. Monitor Urine Color: Urine color can serve as a simple indicator of hydration status. Aim for pale yellow urine, indicating adequate hydration. Dark yellow or amber-colored urine may indicate dehydration and should prompt increased fluid intake.

3. Account for Fluid Losses: Seniors may be at increased risk of dehydration due to factors such as medication side effects, reduced thirst sensation, and age-related changes in kidney function. Consider factors such as weather conditions, physical activity level, and medication use when assessing fluid needs.

4. Include Hydrating Foods: In addition to beverages, certain fruits and vegetables have high water content and contribute to overall hydration. Encourage seniors to consume water-rich foods such as cucumbers, watermelon, strawberries, and lettuce as part of their daily diet.

5. Limit Caffeine and Alcohol: Caffeinated beverages like coffee, tea, and soda can have a diuretic effect, increasing urine production and potentially leading to dehydration if consumed in excess. Similarly, alcohol can dehydrate the body and should be consumed in moderation or avoided, especially for seniors with kidney disease.

Limiting High-Potassium Beverages

For seniors with stage 3 kidney disease, managing potassium intake is crucial to prevent hyperkalemia (elevated potassium levels in the blood), which can be harmful to kidney function and cardiovascular health. Here are some tips for limiting high-potassium beverages:

1. Read Labels: Check the nutrition labels on beverages for their potassium content. Avoid or limit beverages that are high in potassium, such as certain fruit juices, coconut water, and sports drinks.

2. Choose Lower-Potassium Alternatives: Opt for beverages that are lower in potassium, such as diluted fruit juices, herbal teas, and homemade smoothies with low-potassium fruits.

3. Portion Control: If seniors choose to consume higher-potassium beverages occasionally, encourage them to practice portion control and limit their intake to smaller servings to help manage potassium levels.

4. Consult with a Registered Dietitian: Individualized nutrition guidance from a registered dietitian can help seniors with kidney disease navigate their beverage choices while managing their potassium intake within recommended limits.

DINING OUT AND SOCIALIZING

Dining out and socializing can present unique challenges for individuals managing their dietary restrictions, but with careful planning and knowledge, it's possible to enjoy these activities while prioritizing kidney health.

Navigating Restaurant Menus

1. Research and Plan Ahead:

- Encourage seniors to research restaurants beforehand and look for establishments that offer healthier options and are willing to accommodate dietary restrictions.

- Many restaurants now provide their menus online, making it easier for individuals to review options and identify kidney-friendly choices in advance.

2. Understanding Menu Terminology:

- Educate seniors about menu terminology commonly used to indicate dishes that may be suitable for their dietary needs, such as "grilled," "steamed," "baked," or "broiled," which typically signify lower sodium and fat content.

- Advise them to be cautious of terms like "smoked," "marinated," or "crispy," as these may indicate higher sodium or potassium levels.

3. Customizing Orders:

- Encourage seniors to feel comfortable customizing their orders to meet their dietary requirements. They can request modifications such as substituting high-potassium sides with lower-potassium options or asking for sauces and dressings on the side to control sodium intake.

4. Portion Control:

- Remind seniors about the importance of portion control when dining out. Encourage them to consider sharing large entrees or opting for appetizer-sized portions to help manage their sodium, potassium, and phosphorus intake.

5. Communication with Servers:

- Advise seniors to communicate openly with their servers about their dietary restrictions and needs. Many restaurants are willing to accommodate special requests or provide additional information about ingredients upon request.

Hosting Kidney-Friendly Gatherings

1. Menu Planning:

- When hosting gatherings at home, encourage seniors to plan a kidney-friendly menu that considers their guests' dietary restrictions, including low-sodium, low-potassium, and low-phosphorus options.
- Provide a variety of dishes that are flavorful and satisfying without compromising kidney health, such as grilled vegetables, lean proteins, and whole grain salads.

2. Recipe Modifications:

- Offer guidance on modifying traditional recipes to make them kidney-friendly. For example, substituting high-potassium ingredients with lower-potassium alternatives or using herbs and spices to enhance flavor without adding extra salt.

3. Labeling and Communication:

- Clearly label dishes to indicate their nutritional content, particularly highlighting items that may be higher in sodium, potassium, or phosphorus.

- Encourage open communication with guests about dietary restrictions and preferences to ensure everyone feels comfortable and included.

4. Hydration Station:

- Provide a variety of refreshing, kidney-friendly beverages such as infused water, herbal teas, and homemade fruit spritzers to keep guests hydrated without excess sugar or potassium.

Dining Etiquette for Seniors with Kidney Disease

1. Moderation is Key:

- Remind seniors to practice moderation when indulging in restaurant meals or social gatherings. Savoring smaller portions and taking time to enjoy each bite can help prevent overeating and manage nutrient intake.

2. Mindful Eating Practices:

- Encourage seniors to practice mindful eating by paying attention to hunger and fullness cues. Suggest they take breaks between bites, chew slowly, and engage in conversation to prevent mindless overeating.

3. Staying Hydrated:

- Emphasize the importance of staying hydrated, especially when dining out or socializing. Encourage seniors to sip water throughout the meal and limit alcoholic beverages, which can contribute to dehydration.

4. Respecting Dietary Restrictions:

- Remind seniors to assertively communicate their dietary restrictions to hosts, servers, or guests when dining out or attending social gatherings. It's important to prioritize their health needs while still enjoying the social aspect of dining.

5. Gratitude and Appreciation: - Encourage seniors to express gratitude for the effort put into accommodating their dietary needs, whether dining out or attending a social event. Showing appreciation fosters positive relationships and encourages future support.

CONCLUSION

Managing stage 3 kidney disease requires a multifaceted approach that includes medical treatment, lifestyle adjustments, and most importantly, dietary changes. Through this cookbook, we've aimed to provide seniors with stage 3 kidney disease a comprehensive resource filled with delicious and nutritious recipes tailored to their dietary restrictions and nutritional needs.

By incorporating the principles of kidney-friendly eating into your daily routine, you can not only slow the progression of kidney disease but also improve your overall health and quality of life. Remember, small changes can lead to significant improvements, and every meal is an opportunity to nourish your body and support your kidney health.

We encourage you to experiment with the recipes in this cookbook, adapt them to suit your taste preferences, and share them with your loved ones. Together, we can embark on this journey towards better kidney health and enjoy flavorful meals that nourish both body and soul.

Thank you for joining us on this culinary adventure. Here's to good health and happy cooking!